Caregiving at Home

William Leahy, MD
and The Editors of Hartman Publishing

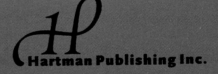

Hartman Publishing Inc.   *hartman*online.com

Albuquerque, NM

Copyright Information

© 2005 by Hartman Publishing Inc. and William Leahy, MD
8529 Indian School Road NE
Albuquerque NM 87112
(505) 291-1274
web: www.hartmanonline.com
e-mail: orders@hartmanonline.com

Publisher's Cataloging-in-Publication
(Provided by Quality Books, Inc.)

Leahy, William.
    Caregiving at home / William Leahy and the editors of
Hartman Publishing.
    p. cm.
    Includes index.
    ISBN 1-888343-90-7

    1. Caregivers--Handbooks, manuals, etc. 2. Home care
services--Handbooks, manuals, etc.   I. Hartman
Publishing. II. Title.

RA645.3.L425 2005   649.8
              QBI05-600010

Notice to the Readers

Though the guidelines and procedures contained in this text are based on consultations with healthcare professionals, they should not be considered absolute recommendations.

The publisher, authors, and editors cannot accept any responsibility for errors or omissions or for any consequences from application of the information in this book and make no warranty, expressed or implied, with respect to the contents of the book. The publisher does not warrant or guarantee any of the products described herein or perform any analysis in connection with any of the product information contained herein.

Even properly performed, not every procedure is safe and appropriate for everyone. Before performing any care procedure listed in this text, consult a physician to learn which procedures are appropriate for your loved one. Ask for a healthcare professional to demonstrate the correct way to do the procedure and adapt these procedures for your loved one's condition.

Internet addresses and telephone numbers listed in this book were correct at press time.

Gender Usage

This textbook utilizes the pronouns "he," "his," "she," and "hers" interchangeably to denote family caregivers and their loved ones.

Credits

Managing Editor
Susan Alvare

Development Editors
Jennifer Plane Hartman
Suzanne Wegner

Cover and Interior Designer
Kirsten Browne

Page Layout
Thaddeus Castillo

Illustration
Thaddeus Castillo

Photography
Art Clifton/Dick Ruddy/Susana Marks

Proofreader
Kristin Calderon

Sales
Gailynn Garberding/Debbie Rinker

Customer Service
Yvonne Gillam/Kim Williams

Acknowledgments

William Leahy, MD became involved with home health aide education both out of an interest in the care his patients received and to give direction and meaning to the lives of young people in his community. After teaching the home health aide program at Bladensburg High School in suburban Maryland, he undertook the project of writing a better book. All royalties from sales of this book fund a foundation formed to support young people studying healthcare careers.

Since 1994 Hartman Publishing has developed educational material for frontline healthcare workers. Nurses are the lifeblood of frontline care, and they have guided each step we've taken. A sincere thank you to the wonderful nurses who have contributed to the material drawn on for this project:

Jetta Fuzy, RN, MS; Julie Grafe, RN, BSN; Betty Wolfe, RN; Susan Cutro, RN; BSN, Anna Blum, RN, MS; Linda Westerman, RN, MN; Delores Pederson, BSN; Charles A. Illian, RN, BSN, CIC; Kathlene Benson, BSN, RN, C

Table of Contents

Table of Procedures

Warning

Even properly performed, not every procedure is safe and appropriate for everyone. Performed incorrectly, they can cause injury to your loved one or yourself. And, some procedures can be dangerous for persons with certain conditions. Before performing any procedure, consult your physician to learn which procedures are appropriate for your loved one. Ask for a healthcare professional to demonstrate the correct way to do the procedure and how to adapt these procedures for your loved one's condition.

Since 1994 our textbooks have helped train home health aides and nursing assistants. Soon thereafter, family caregivers called looking for the same help in understanding the basics of caregiving. ***Caregiving at Home*** is the result of these requests.

Caregiving is amazingly rewarding and important work. At times, it is also exhausting and frustrating.

This book provides a foundation of knowledge to best coordinate a loved one's care and provide the hands-on assistance he or she requires. A section that covers 13 of the most common diseases and conditions among the elderly is included.

Much of the material in this book was originally developed to train certified home health aides and nursing assistants; thus, many of the photographs show uniformed professionals providing care. This information has been used in thousands of successful training programs; it is regularly reviewed and updated to meet the latest medical standards.

Here's how it works:

Color tabs located on the side of every page make finding information simple.

First Steps

Each chapter offers a few "First Steps" to help get you started.

GUIDELINES

Care guidelines are included for over 33 typical problems, including prompts to report subtle changes to a professional caregiver.

Providing foot care

Seventy-two procedures help prepare you for hands-on tasks like bathing and other activities of daily living.

Resources

Concise lists of resources can help provide answers you need. We've limited our resources sections to the most trusted, established, reliable sources to help you quickly find good information.

Tools for organizing medications, holding family meetings, and coordinating care.

Prescribed Medication Schedule

List all medications taken and the times and conditions under which they should be taken.

Time or day	Name of medication	Dosage	How to take

Aging

A primer on aging—what's normal and what's not.

1

Thinking About Home Care

Caring for a family member or loved one in your home can be both challenging and rewarding. This chapter explores these challenges and rewards so you can make informed decisions about caring for a family member at home.

For the person receiving care, the benefits of being in a home environment are significant:

- Most of us feel more comfortable in a private residence than we would in an institutional setting, even if the home in question is not our own.

- Being surrounded by family or other loved ones can combat loneliness (Fig. 1-1).

12

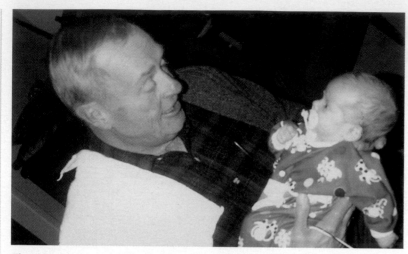

Fig. 1-1. Being surrounded by family can help your loved one combat loneliness.

- Greater independence may be possible in the home (Fig. 1-2).

- Family caregivers provide cost savings.

There are benefits for the caregiver as well, especially the satisfaction of allowing a spouse, parent, or other loved one to recuperate or live out her life in comfort, with dignity and companionship.

Of course, there are difficulties to be faced. For the person receiving care, any move will require adjustment. Any change in health status will

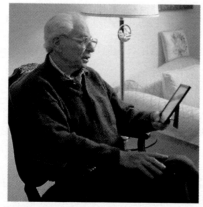

Fig. 1-2. Living in a home environment may allow your loved one more independence than is possible in a facility.

entail changes in relationships with those providing care. It may be difficult for someone to accept help or feel dependent upon a spouse or child when he is used to caring for himself.

For the caregiver, the challenges of providing care in the home are significant:

- Work and family schedules must be modified to allow for caregiving.

- Additional emotional and physical energy must be available.

- The home must be adapted to be safe and practical for your loved one's needs, as well as others in the home.

- Family dynamics will be altered by the change in the household.

- Financial issues will arise (Fig. 1-3).

- Leisure time will be reduced or eliminated.

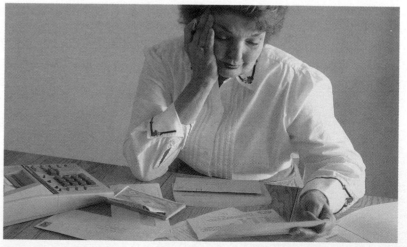

Fig. 1-3. Caring for someone in the home can cause financial difficulties.

Only you can evaluate the challenges and benefits of home care for your particular situation. The considerations listed above provide a starting point for your thoughts. It is a good idea to write down the potential positive and negative impacts, your concerns, and your hopes about providing home care. Consider sharing your thoughts with a person you trust who can help you weigh the pros and cons to make a good decision.

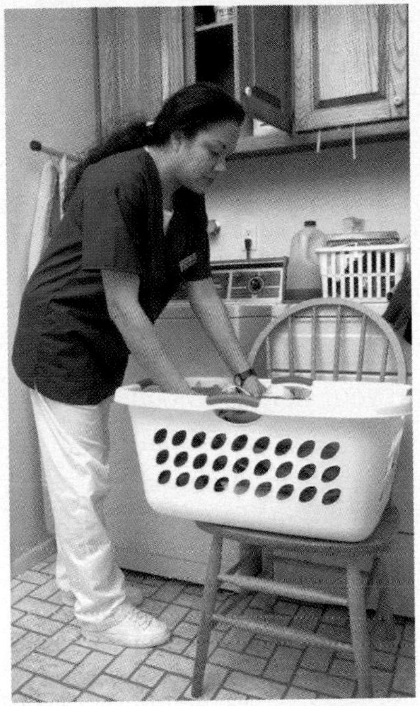

Fig. 1-4. There are many agencies, both paid and volunteer, which can provide assistance for home caregivers.

Available Support

When you are caring for someone in your home, you cannot and should not expect to do everything yourself. There are many sources of support available to you, from adult daycare services for the elderly or disabled to personal grooming or housecleaning services provided by agencies or individuals (Fig. 1-4). Most of these will be listed in the phone book. Many kinds of volunteer help may be available in your community as well, such as church groups, relatives, or friends. Try to accept help when it is offered, and solicit help when it seems to be available. You will be a better caregiver if you take advantage of outside support.

First Steps

Write down the pros and cons of caring for your loved one in your home. Try to separate your emotions from practical considerations as you do this.

Check with your employer about possible benefits for family caregivers. The Family and Medical Leave Act may provide unpaid time off for caregiving. Visit www.benefitscheckup.org to determine what kind of financial benefits your loved one is eligible to receive. Created by the National Council on the Aging (NCOA) this free, easy-to-use website helps older Americans determine their eligibility for a wide range of public assistance programs. It compares the information you give with eligibility requirements for Social Security, Medicaid, food stamps, weatherization, in-home services, pharmacy programs, and state programs. A printable report of programs and enrollment information is available.

Find out as much as you can about your loved one's special needs and abilities and how they will affect daily life for you and other members of the household.

Locate resources in your area that will be able to help you as a caregiver. A good resource to check with is the Eldercare Locator at www.eldercare.gov, 1-800-677-1116.

Here are some options to explore for finding help in your community:

Area Agency on Aging: This is a great place to start, as they will have details about all of the services that follow. Services may include information and referrals regarding health insurance, transportation, meal delivery services, and homemaker services. To find Area Agencies on Aging across the country, call the Eldercare Locator at 1-800-677-1116.

Senior centers or community centers may offer caregiver support groups, adult daycare or respite care.

Meals on Wheels is a meal delivery service for homebound people (Fig. 1-5).

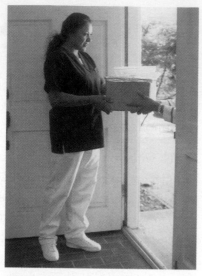

Fig. 1-5. Meals on Wheels is a meal delivery service for people who cannot leave home.

Hospitals or nursing homes may offer caregiver support groups or adult daycare or respite care.

The Alzheimer's Association, The American Cancer Society, or other disease-specific organizations may offer support groups or other services.

County Health Nurse: Local or county departments of health or human services sometimes offer eldercare programs.

Hospices provide services for patients who have fewer than six month to live.

Home health agencies offer personal and home health services, such as help with bathing, dressing, feeding and meal preparation on an hourly fee basis. Clients with Medicare who are homebound may qualify for reimbursement of some home health expenses (Fig. 1-6).

Faith-based groups, including churches, temples, or other groups, may offer volunteers to visit homebound patients, provide respite care, drive patients to appointments, prepare meals or perform household tasks. Contact large congregations in your neighborhood and ask about their social ministries, neighborhood outreach, or eldercare programs.

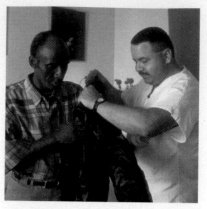

Fig. 1-6. People who are eligible for Medicare may qualify for some reimbursement of home care expenses.

Accepting Help

Sometimes caregivers feel it is simpler to do everything themselves than to accept or solicit help from others. It may indeed be simpler, but it will also be more tiring. No one can do everything that is required of a caregiver in the home without accepting some help. To preserve your physical, mental, and emotional health, you must give yourself a break and find ways to share the duties of caregiving.

If your loved one resists accepting care from anyone but you, you may have to be creative to get a break for yourself. Perhaps you can let someone else do the cooking, cleaning, and shopping while you provide personal care such as bathing and dressing (Fig. 1-7). Somehow you will need to find relief for yourself if you are to continue as a loving, reliable caregiver.

Often friends and neighbors offer to help but do not know what to do. Help them to help you. Give them specific ideas of things they can do for you or your loved one. The list below includes specific ways others can help you. Tailor the list to your specific situation; add other things needed and keep it available for friends and neighbors who want to help.

1. Sit with my loved one so I can run an errand, take a nap, read a book, go to a movie, or take a walk to clear my head.

2. Help with errands that we need done, for example, doing the grocery shopping.

3. Prepare a meal and bring it over in dishes that do not need to be returned. Things that can be frozen are always good, as they provide flexibility.

4. Offer to take my loved one out as appropriate (Fig. 1-8). Be prepared to walk slowly or push the wheelchair. If you can find a meeting, program

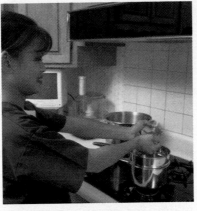

Fig. 1-7. Even if your loved one prefers to have care only from you, there are plenty of opportunities for others to help out around the home.

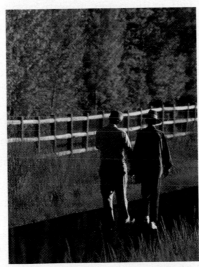

Fig. 1-8. If appropriate, ask a friend or family member to take your loved one out.

or concert that might be appropriate and of interest, invite him there.

5. Write down the times you are available and what you are prepared to do so I can call you. For example: Thursday evenings and Saturday afternoons I can run errands, sit with your loved one, or bring over dinners.

6. Take my car to get the oil changed and fill it with gas. Run it through the car wash to give us a real treat.

7. Offer to bring over your own cleaning supplies and clean a room or two or mop the kitchen floor.

8. Ask if there is laundry to be done and do it. Visit with us while the loads wash and dry.

9. Bring over something special to interest my loved one: family photos or videos, a musical instrument you can play, or a simple craft project to do together (Fig. 1-9).

10. Take me out, if I can get away, for a meal, a movie, a massage, or just some time away from the responsibilities at home.

11. Offer to mow the lawn, balance the checkbook, fill out insurance forms, shop for gifts, pay bills, answer correspondence, or do anything else I cannot find the time or energy to do.

12. Be positive! Tell me I'm doing a good job. Give us

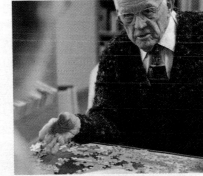

Fig. 1-9. Ask friends to bring over pleasant things to share with your loved one.

hugs if that feels right. Bring silly jokes to share. You never know what can lift spirits.

13. Be sensitive. Listen to what my words and my body language are telling you. Offer to come back another time if things seem strained.

If you have access to the Internet, there are several websites intended for caregivers that may be of interest to you (Fig. 1-10). Phone numbers are included so you can call for information if you do not have Internet access. More agencies and websites are located at the end of the chapter in the "Resources" section.

Family Caregiver Alliance
www.caregiver.org
800-445-8106

National Family Caregiver Association
www.thefamilycaregiver.org

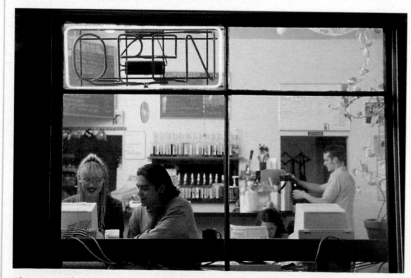

Fig. 1-10. The Internet is a good source of information for caregivers.

800-896-3650
Membership in this organization is free for any family caregiver.

Alternatives to Home Care

As you think about providing home care, it is helpful to know what other options exist. Your ability to provide care may change with personal circumstances, or your loved one's needs may change, necessitating a change in living and care arrangements. For example, many families caring for a person with dementia find there is a point where it is no longer physically safe to keep the person at home; wandering, aggression, and physical outbursts may require the person to be moved to a facility designed for those suffering from dementia. If you have found the best possible way to meet your loved one's needs, as well as the needs of your family, then you have succeeded as a caregiver, whether the solution is care in the home or care in a facility.

Adult Daycare

Adult daycare is given at a facility during daytime work hours. Generally, adult daycare cares for people who need some help but are not seriously ill or disabled. Adult daycare centers give different levels of care. Adult daycare can also provide a break for spouses and family members.

Semi-Independent Living Arrangements

Retirement homes, senior apartments, homes for the elderly, and condominium communities are designed for people who can manage with some assistance. These arrangements may be appealing if you or your loved one wants more privacy or space than is available in your home. Group activities may also be available. These living accommodations are usually not designed for the frail elderly or those needing daily assistance with bathing, dressing, and eating.

Assisted Living Facilities

This growing category usually describes a group of apartments where meals and housekeeping are included in the rent. Twenty-four-hour emergency medical help may be available; for an additional fee, assistance can be arranged for everything from bathing to dressing to trips to the doctor. The regulations governing these facilities vary widely from state to state, so the level of care provided must be determined on an individual basis. These facilities can be expensive and are usually not covered by insurance or Medicare.

Continuing Care Retirement Facilities

These providers offer a lifetime contract for care in exchange for a substantial entrance fee plus monthly fees that depend on the care required. For example, a person may enter at age 65 able to live independently in an apartment. Later he moves to an assisted living unit with meals provided until he finally needs skilled nursing care in a specialized unit.

Nursing Homes or Skilled Nursing Facilities

These facilities provide daily care, ranging from help with dressing, bathing, and eating to medication monitoring, oxy-

gen therapy, IV therapy, or skilled nursing care. These facilities provide long-term care and assist those with chronic conditions (Fig. 1-11).

Specialized Facilities for Dementia

Some nursing homes and assisted living facilities have specialized wings or separate buildings dedicated to the housing and care of people with dementia. These are secure facilities which may allow residents to wander without leaving the safety of the facility. These facilities have staff and programs that are specifically geared to meeting the needs of residents with dementia.

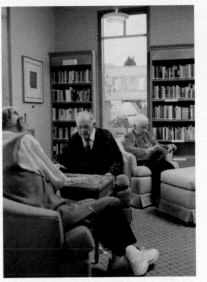

Fig. 1-11. Nursing homes offer 24-hour skilled care for people with a variety of needs.

There may also be other options in your community to help care for the elderly or infirm. Keep your mind open to various options so that as your loved one's needs change, you are prepared to adapt your arrangement as necessary.

Financial and Legal Issues

Managing the finances of a person who is ill or dying is complicated. The regulations governing Medicare and Medicaid and the benefits from Social Security or from private insurers change often and vary with individual situations. Thus it is difficult to present a general guide to dealing with these financial issues.

However, a basic understanding of what these programs are can help. Further, there are some rules for managing finances that will apply across the board.

Medicare

Medicare is the federal insurance program created in 1965 to provide healthcare for the elderly and disabled. Medicare Part A, or Hospital Insurance, is free for eligible citizens. It is financed through the Social Security or FICA tax paid by workers and employers. Medicare Part A helps cover the cost of stays in the hospital, surgery and recovery, lab work, X-rays, and some rehabilitation (Fig. 1-12). Currently, Medicare Part A pays for some care in a nursing home following a hospital stay. However, Medicare does not cover continuing care in a nursing facility, nor does Medicare currently cover the costs of home health care unless the patient is officially homebound and in need of some skilled nursing services. Some assistance with prescription drugs is available under the Medicare Prescription Drug Improvement and

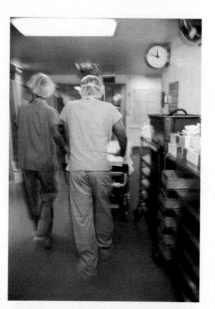

Fig. 1-12. Medicare Part A pays for some hospital and surgery expenses.

Modernization Act of 2003. To find out if your loved one is eligible, visit www.medicare.gov. Check back with the site often; this is new legislation and there are likely to be changes.

Medicare Part B, or Medical Insurance, deducts monthly premiums from the Social Security checks of those who enroll. Part B covers some costs of doctor's visits and other medical expenses.

Call the Medicare Hotline (1-800-MEDICARE, or 1-800-633-4227) for more information and to obtain brochures explaining current Medicare benefits and procedures.

Medicaid

Also established in 1965, Medicaid is a joint federal-state program intended to help finance health care for the poor and the long-term care needs of people impoverished by medical expenses. People of any age whose income falls below a certain level can be eligible for Medicaid coverage. People in need of long-term care, whether at home or in a facility, can become eligible for Medicaid assistance after their own assets have been depleted (Fig. 1-13).

Private Long-Term Care Insurance

More insurers are offering long-term care policies in response to consumer fears of asset depletion and confinement to substandard long-term care facilities. People who have substantial assets to protect and a family history of needing long-term care as they age may wish to consider private long-term care insurance. To qualify, applicants must be in good general physical and mental health. Premiums may be high, and benefits vary

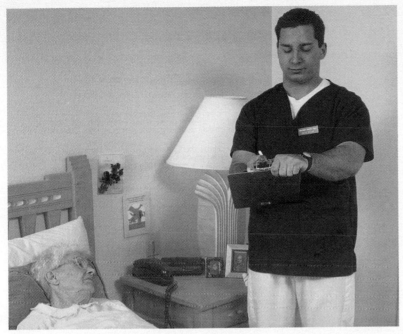

Fig. 1-13. Some people in need of long-term care may be eligible for benefits from Medicaid.

greatly. Deal with reputable agents only; check insurers' ratings. Understand the benefits and restrictions clearly before making a commitment to purchase a policy.

GUIDELINES
Handling Finances

Keep all financial records. Make notes of phone calls, with whom you spoke, the date, and what you were told.

Separate the papers regarding the person you are caring for from your own financial papers. Create a file box, even just a cardboard box, where you can keep your loved one's records.

Ask questions. Healthcare billing can be confusing. Be sure you understand what you are paying for, how much you are being reimbursed, and when another payment is due.

Be persistent. Follow up with the business office, the claims department, or the Medicare office when you need something resolved. Put your concerns in writing if that makes it easier to communicate and keep records.

Ask for help. There may be someone among your friends or relatives who is more comfortable dealing with finances than caregiving. Helping you pay the bills, balance the checkbook, file insurance claims, or keep medical records could be a way for that person to lighten your burden.

Other Legal Issues

Last Will and Testament

Everyone should have a will prepared and signed. If this has not been done, it should be done soon. A simple will can be prepared using prewritten legal forms purchased at an office supply store. An attorney should handle any complicated situations.

Power of Attorney

Creating a Power of Attorney gives authority to a designated party to make financial and legal decisions for someone else. Execute a new Power of Attorney every few years so that the intention to delegate authority is clearly established.

Advance Directives

Various documents can be executed to establish a person's instructions for health care at the end of life or in critical care situations. Living Wills, Health Care Proxies, and Do Not Resuscitate Orders are all ways of clarifying a person's wishes or designating someone to make decisions in the event of incapacitation (Fig. 1-14). The forms for these directives vary but are generally easy to obtain from doctors, hospitals or nursing homes. You can also download your state's packages/forms at www.choices.org. Fill them out and have them signed and witnessed right away; update them periodically.

Resources

The official U.S. government site for Medicare has links for comparing nursing homes, home health agencies, and dialysis centers in your area.

Centers for Medicare & Medicaid Services (CMS)
7500 Security Boulevard
Baltimore MD 21244-1850
www.medicare.gov

FirstGov.gov is a government site with information to help seniors conduct business with federal agencies more quickly and easily.

FirstGov.gov for Seniors
U.S. General Services Administration
1800 F Street NW
Washington, DC 20405
800-FED-INFO (800-333-4636)
www.seniors.gov

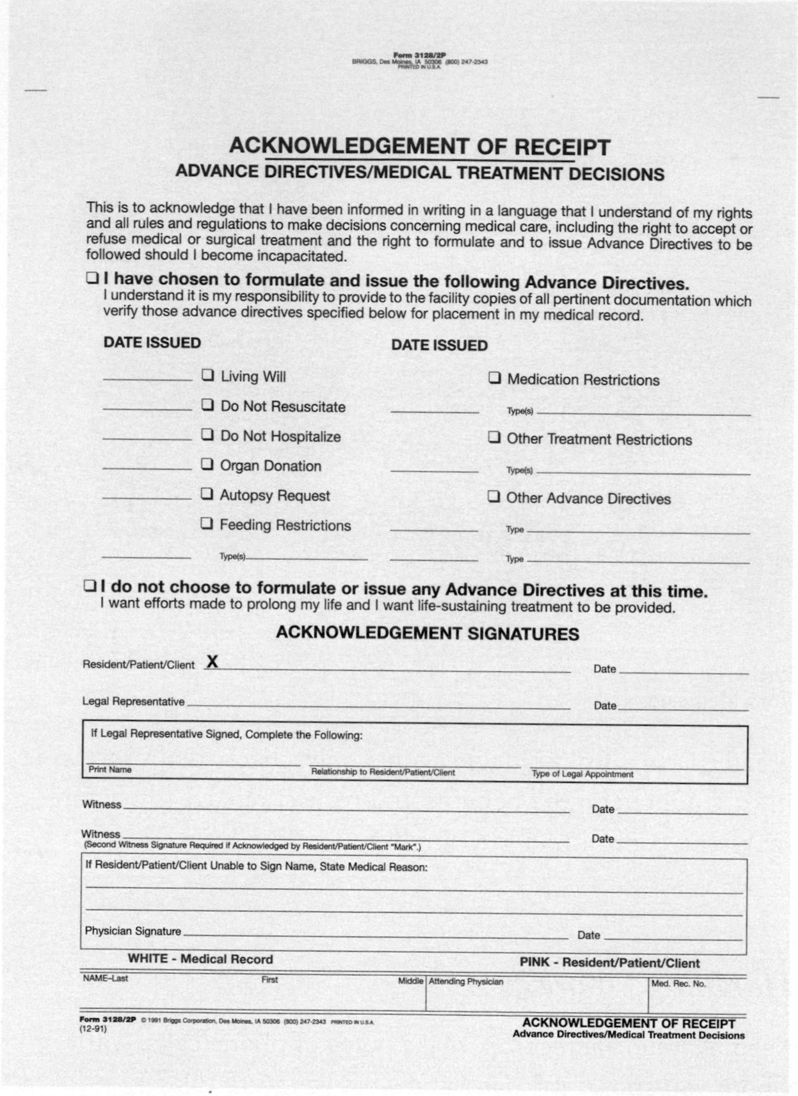

Form 3128/2P
BRIGGS, Des Moines, IA 50306 (800) 247-2343
PRINTED IN U.S.A.

ACKNOWLEDGEMENT OF RECEIPT
ADVANCE DIRECTIVES/MEDICAL TREATMENT DECISIONS

This is to acknowledge that I have been informed in writing in a language that I understand of my rights and all rules and regulations to make decisions concerning medical care, including the right to accept or refuse medical or surgical treatment and the right to formulate and to issue Advance Directives to be followed should I become incapacitated.

❑ **I have chosen to formulate and issue the following Advance Directives.**
I understand it is my responsibility to provide to the facility copies of all pertinent documentation which verify those advance directives specified below for placement in my medical record.

DATE ISSUED		DATE ISSUED	
________	❑ Living Will		❑ Medication Restrictions
________	❑ Do Not Resuscitate	________	Type(s) ________
________	❑ Do Not Hospitalize		❑ Other Treatment Restrictions
________	❑ Organ Donation	________	Type(s) ________
________	❑ Autopsy Request		❑ Other Advance Directives
	❑ Feeding Restrictions	________	Type ________
________	Type(s) ________	________	Type ________

❑ **I do not choose to formulate or issue any Advance Directives at this time.**
I want efforts made to prolong my life and I want life-sustaining treatment to be provided.

ACKNOWLEDGEMENT SIGNATURES

Resident/Patient/Client X ________ Date ________

Legal Representative ________ Date ________

If Legal Representative Signed, Complete the Following:
Print Name ________ Relationship to Resident/Patient/Client ________ Type of Legal Appointment ________

Witness ________ Date ________

Witness ________ Date ________
(Second Witness Signature Required if Acknowledged by Resident/Patient/Client "Mark".)

If Resident/Patient/Client Unable to Sign Name, State Medical Reason:

Physician Signature ________ Date ________

WHITE - Medical Record **PINK - Resident/Patient/Client**

NAME–Last First Middle | Attending Physician | Med. Rec. No.

Form 3128/2P © 1991 Briggs Corporation, Des Moines, IA 50306 (800) 247-2343 PRINTED IN U.S.A. (12-91)

ACKNOWLEDGEMENT OF RECEIPT
Advance Directives/Medical Treatment Decisions

Fig. 1-14. Advance directives let you know a person's wishes regarding treatment if he or she should become incapacitated. (Reprinted with permission of Briggs Corporation, 800-247-2343)

The Administration on Aging website educates older people and caregivers about benefits and services that can help them.

The U.S. Administration on Aging
Washington, DC 20201
202-619-0724
www.aoa.dhhs.gov

The American Association of Retired Persons (AARP) website has information, education, advocacy, and community information for people over 50.

American Association of Retired Persons (AARP)
601 E. Street NW
Washington, DC 20049
888-OUR-AARP (888-687-2277)
www.AARP.org

The Healthy Aging for Older Adults website sponsored by the National Center for Chronic Disease Prevention and Health Promotion provides information on a wide range of topics including the following: health-related behaviors, chronic diseases, infectious diseases, immunizations for adults, and injuries among older adults.

National Center for Chronic Disease Prevention and Health Promotion: Healthy Aging for Older Adults
1600 Clifton Rd
Atlanta, GA 30333
404-639-3311
www.cdc.gov/aging

NOTE: In the United States every state regulates healthcare facilities differently. In your state, private home health agencies may not be formally regulated. The same holds true for assisted living homes and adult foster homes. Quality can vary widely. We direct you to local resources because they are the BEST source of up-to-date information in your community. Make contacting them a priority.

Communication

Communication—talking, listening, and exchanging information—is at the heart of caregiving. Effective communication will allow you to understand your loved one's needs, express your concerns to the doctor, and ask for the help you need from others. Communication becomes more difficult when people are tired, in pain, frustrated, or depressed. It is easy to become distracted, confused, or intimidated in a doctor's office or on the phone with an insurance representative. When communication breaks down, the misunderstandings that arise can range from inconvenient to disastrous. By keeping a few basic communication principles in mind, you can keep the flow of information open with your family and with the care team.

First Steps

Ascertain any special needs that your loved one has that might affect communication. Does he have hearing, vision, or speech impairments? Is there dementia or confusion? Talk with any former caregivers to get an idea of what kind of communication has been effective for them. Also talk with healthcare professionals in the field relating to your loved one's impairment for communication strategies. Be prepared to adjust communication strategies as his condition changes.

Talk to your loved one about the care she is receiving. Find out how she feels about the members of the care team, the care plan, and how it is being implemented. Ask how she has responded to treatments and how they have affected the quality of her life. Find out if there are any needs that she has that are not being met to her satisfaction.

Make consultation appointments with all of your loved one's doctors to find out the details of the care plan. Get as much information about treatment and expected outcomes as you can; it is helpful to ask for written information or even take a tape recorder with you to the consultation.

Communication Basics

Communication is the process that we use to send and receive messages and exchange information with other people. We communicate using signs and symbols, including words, drawings, and pictures, and also by behavior and gestures. The simplest form of communication takes place between two

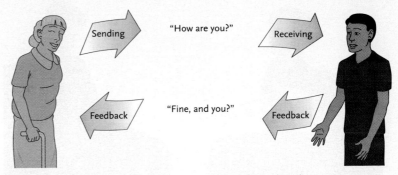

Fig. 2-1. The simplest form of communication takes place between two people.

people—a sender and a receiver (Fig. 2-1). These two constantly switch roles as communication takes place. The next step, providing feedback, occurs when the receiver repeats or responds to the sender's message, letting the sender know that the message was received and understood. During a conversation, this three-step process is usually repeated over and over.

Communication can be either verbal or nonverbal, that is, with or without words. Nodding your head instead of saying "yes" is nonverbal communication. The tone or emphasis we give to words is also nonverbal communication. Consider the difference between "I'll be right there, Mother!" and "I'll *be* right *there*, Mother!"

Body language is a form of nonverbal communication. Movements, facial expressions, and posture can express different attitudes or emotions, including sadness, happiness, anger, and pain. Just as when speaking, we send messages with our body language that other people receive and interpret. For example, slouching in a chair and sitting erect send two different messages—you are bored, tired or hostile versus you are interested and respectful (Fig. 2-2).

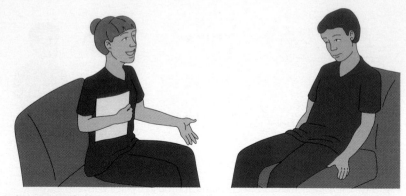

Fig. 2-2. Body language is a nonverbal form of communication. The person on the right does not seem to be as interested in the conversation as the person on the left.

Sometimes people send one message verbally and a very different one nonverbally. Nonverbal communication often tells us how someone is feeling, despite what he or she is saying. Your loved one may tell you, "I'm feeling a little better," but stay in bed and stare blankly at the wall. Such nonverbal clues can tell you he may be depressed. You may need to say something like, "Dad, you don't seem to be feeling better. You seem to be feeling down today." This could open the door for verbal communication and allow him to express his feelings, or at least allow you to acknowledge what he is feeling.

Barriers to Communication

Communication can be blocked or disrupted in many ways (Fig. 2-3). The following are some barriers to communication and ways to avoid them:

- **Your loved one does not hear or understand what you say.** Speak clearly, and check that any hearing aid is being worn and is working.

- **You do not hear or understand what she is telling you.** Ask her to repeat what she has said. Rephrase the message in your own words to make sure you have understood. Use pictures or gestures.

- **The meaning of words or terms is not clear.** Clarify meanings. Use simple words and avoid medical terminology.

- **Using slang confuses the message.** Avoid using slang words or expressions.

- **Using clichés makes your message meaningless.** Instead of using a cliché, such as "Everything will be all right," listen to what is really being said. Then respond accordingly. For example, "I understand you are worried about this doctor's appointment. How could I make it go more smoothly for you?"

- **Asking "why" makes your loved one defensive.** When someone makes a statement such as "I don't want to go for a walk today," responding by asking "Why?" or "Why not?" can elicit an angry response. Instead, try asking, "Are you feeling tired right now?" or "Is there something else you'd like to do first?" This allows you to open up a conversation that is more helpful in resolving the question.

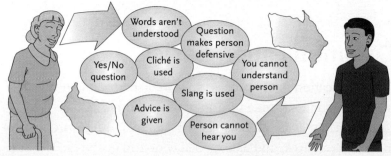

Fig. 2-3. There are many obstacles that can disrupt communication.

- **Yes/no answers end a conversation.** Unless you are seeking direct information, ask open-ended questions that need more than a "yes" or "no" answer. For example, ask, "What kinds of things would you like to do when people come over?" instead of, "Do you want to play cards when people come to visit?"

Accurate and Complete Communication

In addition to avoiding barriers to communication, these positive techniques will help you send and receive clear, complete messages.

Be a good listener. Allow the other person to express her ideas completely. When she is finished, restate the message in your own words to make sure you have understood (Fig. 2-4).

Provide feedback as you listen. Active listening involves focusing on the message and providing feedback. Offering general but leading responses such as "Oh?" or "Go on," or "Hmm," provides feedback and encourages the sender to expand the message. Other phrases, such as "Oh, really?" or "Tell me more," can also be used.

Bring up topics of concern. If you know a topic that may be of concern, raise it in a general, non-threatening way.

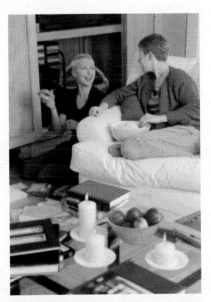

Fig. 2-4. Active listening is an important step in communication.

This allows the other person to decide whether or not they wish to discuss it. For example, you might say, "Mom, you seemed upset after we saw the doctor yesterday." Or, "Mom, you're awfully quiet this morning. Is something on your mind?"

Let some pauses happen. Use silence to allow the other person to gather her thoughts or decide to convey another message. Silence indicates that you are open to receiving messages.

Ask for more. When your loved one reports feelings, events, or symptoms, restate what you have heard to clarify. Ask if there is more he or she can tell you.

Communication and Special Needs

If your loved one has hearing loss, impaired vision, impaired speech, memory loss, confusion, or dementia, communication is more difficult. However, there are ways to address these challenges.

Hearing Impairment

Many people gradually lose their acuity of hearing with age. Sometimes it is a result of an accident, illness, or disease. Many people experience sudden or significant hearing loss or deafness. You may be used to speaking more loudly, slowly or distinctly with your loved one. You may need to model these techniques for other family members or even suggest directly, "Dad will be able to hear you better if you sit facing him, speak slowly, and raise your voice a bit." (Fig. 2-5).

Hearing aids can make a real difference and should be used, maintained, and replaced as needed. Even if it may be the end

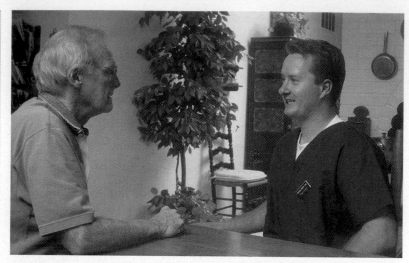

Fig. 2-5. When speaking to a person with hearing impairment, face them directly and speak slowly and clearly.

of life, quality of life is important. Being able to hear and communicate can contribute greatly to quality of life.

When communicating with a person with a hearing impairment, try to reduce the noise in the area you are in; closing doors may help. Make sure you have the person's attention before speaking. Lower the pitch of your voice and do not shout. Use short sentences and simple words, and try to avoid sudden changes of topic.

For those with significant hearing loss, the use of pictures, gestures and signs will enhance communication. You can find photos in magazines or catalogs of common food choices or activity options to make it easier to suggest possibilities to your loved one. She can respond with speech or by pointing. Consider keeping a pad and pencil or a dry-erase board and marker handy to jot down questions or words that are hard for either of you to express.

Vision Impairment

Like hearing, vision often deteriorates with age. Vision also contributes greatly to quality of life. Glasses should be used, maintained and replaced as needed (Fig. 2-6). In the case of more significant loss of sight, greater adaptations can be made. Many special aids, such as clocks or watches that "speak" the time when a button is pressed, or books on tape or in large print, are available. Even little things, like a pad of paper with extra dark rules that allow a person with limited sight to write in straight lines, can make a difference.

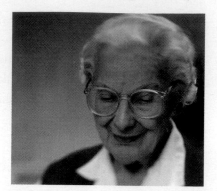

Fig. 2-6. Glasses should be used and cared for as needed.

If your loved one has impaired vision, always identify yourself when you enter the room. Provide good lighting. It may be helpful to use the face of an imaginary clock to describe the position of objects in the room (Fig. 2-7). Do not move furniture without letting him know. Use large clocks, clocks that chime, or radios to help keep track of time. Let him know when you are leaving the room.

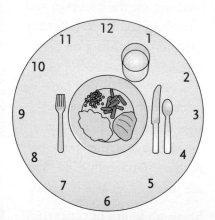

Fig. 2-7. Using the face of an imaginary clock is a good way to describe the position of objects to a visually impaired person.

Impaired Speech

Speech loss or impairment is a common result of stroke. If your loved one has suffered a stroke or brain damage that affects his speech, he may be receiving therapy to improve speech function. Meanwhile, you can communicate using signs and gestures, pencil and paper, and visual aids such as photos or drawings of often-used items. Coping with speech loss is frustrating, and relearning speech is a long and difficult process. Your loved one will need a lot of patience and encouragement from those around him.

If your loved one has impaired speech, keep any questions simple; phrase them so that they can be answered with a "yes" or "no" when possible. Agree on signals, such as shaking the head or raising a finger, to indicate "yes" or "no." If she can write, use a pencil and paper; a thick handle or tape around the handle of a pencil may make writing easier. Use pictures, gestures, or pointing. Use communication boards or special cards to aid communication (see chapter 7).

Memory Loss, Confusion, Dementia

Whatever the cause, memory loss, confusion and dementia make communication difficult. Your loved one may or may not be aware that he is confused or that he has already asked you the same question many times. The more patient and the calmer you are, the better chance you will have of getting through to him. Frustration and agitation will only distract and upset him.

- Always approach your loved one from the front to avoid startling him. Speak quietly and slowly in a low, calm voice, with little background noise and distraction (Fig. 2-8). Try to see and hear yourself as your loved one sees and hears you. Check your body language to make sure you do not appear hurried or impatient.

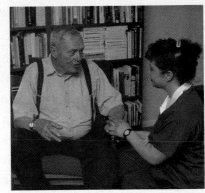

Fig. 2-8. If your loved one is confused, speak to him slowly and clearly and avoid startling him.

- Repeat yourself using the same words or phrases as often as needed. Repetition can be soothing for a person who has dementia or is confused. Ask him to repeat your words to make sure you have been understood. Keep messages simple. Break complex tasks into smaller, simpler ones. Note which communication methods are effective and continue to use them.

- Watch for nonverbal cues as the ability to speak lessens. Use pictures and gestures to communicate. Sometimes nonverbal communication is more effective. You could label the door to the bathroom, for example, with a drawing of a toilet and shower. When speaking, combine verbal and nonverbal communication (Fig. 2-9). For example,

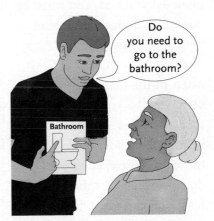

Fig. 2-9. Combining verbal and nonverbal communication can help make your message clearer.

say, "Aunt Jean, it's time to get dressed now," and hold up her clothes as you speak.

- If your loved one is upset but cannot explain why, offer comfort with a hug or a smile. Touch, smiles, and laughter will be understood much longer than spoken or written language. Try to distract him. Verbal communication may be frustrating for him at this time. Assume that your loved one can understand more than he can express. Do not talk about him with others as though he were not there.

Communication with Medical Professionals

Communication with the care team is equally important as communication with your loved one and within your family. Do not hesitate to take an active role in the care of your loved one. You, as caregiver, must understand what plan of care has been established. You must be able to send clear and accurate messages about the state of your loved one's health. As a family caregiver, you are often in the best position to observe changes in symptoms, abilities, or general health. The more clearly these are conveyed to the doctor, nurse, or other professional caregiver, the better care they will provide (Fig. 2-10).

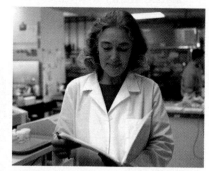

Fig. 2-10. As the primary caregiver, you will be the best person to communicate observations about your loved one's health to the doctor and other members of the care team.

Planning your communication in advance and writing notes will help you get all necessary information across and ensure that all of your questions are answered. Be polite and focus on the information that you need to send and receive rather than any frustrations you may have. While the experience of visiting a doctor's office may be frustrating, it is more important to get the information you need than to express your aggravation.

Terminology and Abbreviations

The medical profession has a great deal of terminology and many abbreviations that are used for communication. Although you are not being trained as a medical worker, it may be useful for you to be aware of some of the most common terms and abbreviations.

Common Abbreviations	
ā	before
abd	abdomen
ac, AC	before meals
ad lib	as desired
am	morning
amb	ambulate
AP	apical pulse
b.i.d., bid	twice daily
BM, B.M.	bowel movement
BP	blood pressure
c̄	with

C	Celsius degree
c/o	complains of
CHF	congestive heart failure
CPR	cardiopulmonary resuscitation
dx or DX	diagnosis
F	Fahrenheit degree
FBS	fasting blood sugar
ft	foot
FWB	full weight-bearing
GI	gastrointestinal
H_2O	water
hr.	hour
I&O	intake and output
NKDA	no known drug allergies
NPO	nothing by mouth
NWB	absolutely no weight on leg
O_2	oxygen
OOB	out of bed
OD	right eye
OS	left eye
p	pulse
p̄	after
p.c., pc	after meals
po	by mouth
PRN	as necessary

PWB	partial weight-bearing
q	every
q.i.d., qid	four times a day
qs	quantity sufficient
R	respirations
ROM	range of motion
s̄	without
SOB	shortness of breath
stat	at once
t.i.d., tid	three times a day
TPR	temperature, pulse, respiration
VS	vital signs
w/c	wheelchair

Observing and Reporting

As a family caregiver, you probably spend more hours with your loved one than anyone else does. You are in an excellent position to observe and report on his condition, including any changes, occurrences, or new symptoms.

Any of the following should be reported immediately to the doctor or home health agency. You may also need to call 911 or go to an emergency room for emergency assistance.

- Fall

- Chest pain

- Severe headache

- Difficulty breathing

- Abnormal pulse, respiration, or blood pressure

- Change in mental status, e.g. confusion

- Sudden weakness or inability to move

- High fever

- Loss of consciousness

- Change in level of consciousness, e.g. confusion

- Bleeding

Less urgent conditions should also be reported. These include:

- Loss of appetite or weight loss

- Rash

- Difficulty sleeping

- Coughing or other respiratory signs

- Persistent pain

- Change in bowel or bladder habits

- Weakness or fatigue

- Nausea

- Depression, withdrawal

Use your common sense when observing and reporting changes to the doctor or nurse. You should not try to diagnose the problem, nor should you try to decide if a complaint is important or trivial. If in doubt, report it.

Always gather your information and write notes before calling the doctor or nurse (Fig. 2-11). Place your call in a quiet room with no distractions. Plan out what you will say in advance; writing notes is a good way to help you remember. If you have to leave a message, make it brief, complete and clear. If someone will call you back, keep the notes by the phone or in your pocket so you can easily find them. Write your observations, when you first noticed them, and any supporting details

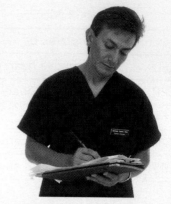

Fig. 2-11. Writing notes before a visit to the doctor will help you make the most of this time.

such as the presence of fever. Always be prepared to give the patient's name, date of birth, social security number, and insurance, Medicare or Medicaid information.

At right is an example of notes made for a call to report concerns about nausea, loss of appetite, and weakness (Fig. 2-12).

Communicating at a Doctor's Visit

All the basic principles of good communication apply when you communicate with the doctor. However, because doctor's visits can be rushed and stressful, it is helpful to have a strategy for improving communication in the doctor's office.

Nauseous since Saturday, hasn't eaten a full meal in 48 hours.

Will only take broth and saltines.

Hasn't left bed except for bathroom - says she is too tired.

No vomiting or fever.

Fig. 2-12.

The following is taken in part from a guide published by the National Family Caregivers Association:

1. Write down questions so you won't forget what you want to ask. You might even want to fax your questions to the doctor in advance to give her a chance to see them in writing.

2. Be clear and concise in speaking to the doctor. Try not to ramble. If you need to give the history of an illness or condition, write down the essential facts beforehand. It is a good idea to tell the doctor what you and your loved one expect and hope for from treatment.

3. If you have many things to discuss, make a consultation appointment so the doctor can allow enough time to meet with you without being rushed.

4. Ask for written copies of the information that you are given, or carry a small tape recorder with you so that you will not have to try to remember everything.

5. If the doctor instructs you to administer treatment you are incapable of or uncomfortable with, let her know.

6. Find out as much as you can about any tests or procedures recommended. What are the benefits and risks? Will it be painful? What are the risks associated with not having the test or procedure done? How will it affect the abilities and quality of life of your loved one in the future?

7. If you have doubts about a treatment or procedure the doctor recommends, do not hesitate to get a second opinion.

8. Learn about your loved one's disease or disability. There are often good resources at the library or on the Internet. You can also use the resources in each chapter of this book.

9. Learn the routine at your doctor's office and/or the hospital. Make the system work for you, not against you (Fig. 2-13).

10. Recognize that not all questions have answers, especially those beginning with "why."

11. Separate your anger and your sense of powerlessness about not being able to cure your loved one from your feelings about the doctor. Remember you are both on the same side.

12. Appreciate what the doctor is doing and say thank you.

Good communication is the basis of good teamwork between you as caregiver, your loved one, and the team of medical professionals providing care.

When to Think About Changing Doctors

Medicine is perhaps the most respected profession in our society, and for good reason—a competent doctor can change or

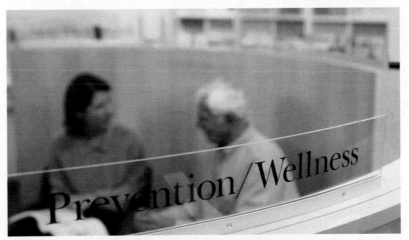

Fig. 2-13. Learning office routines can make doctor visits easier.

save a patient's life. But it is helpful to remember that medicine is also a service profession; you and your loved one can change doctors at any time that you choose. While it is not a good idea to change doctors repeatedly or whimsically as it prevents developing a solid relationship, if you feel your doctor is not right for your loved one, do not hesitate to seek another. The following are some reasons that you might consider changing doctors:

1. The doctor does not seem to listen to your loved one's concerns; she interrupts or is rude or dismissive.

2. The level of care is not satisfactory; the expected response is not achieved on most occasions or the doctor does not seem to know much about your loved one's specific conditions.

3. The doctor does not respond to questions and concerns, or becomes defensive when questions are asked.

4. The doctor is not willing to coordinate care with other doctors or does not adjust treatment to enmesh with other care your loved one is receiving.

5. The doctor refuses to acknowledge mistakes.

6. The doctor becomes defensive or irritated when you choose to seek a second opinion.

7. It is difficult to get an appointment within a reasonable amount of time for a new complaint.

8. The doctor refuses to refer your loved one to a specialist when necessary.

9. The doctor does not satisfactorily explain his reasons for ordering tests, treatments or surgery.

10. The doctor fails to tell you of potential results of treatment or surgery, such as side effects or potential loss of function or change in quality of life.

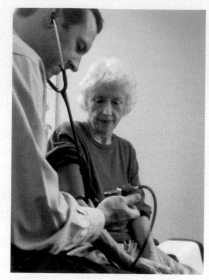

Fig. 2-14. A doctor who is certified in geriatrics may better understand the needs of an older adult.

If at some point you are seeking a new physician, you may want to get a doctor certified in geriatrics. Some internists and general practitioners have extra training regarding the needs and treatments of older adults (Fig. 2-14). Such a physician will be in a better position to understand the multiple conditions and medications your loved one is living with and the effects of aging on the body.

Resources

The American Foundation for the Blind is dedicated to promoting employment, independent living, literacy and technology for those who are visually impaired.

American Foundation for the Blind
11 Penn Plaza, Suite 300
New York, NY 10001
Tel: 212-502-7600
Fax: 212-502-7777
www.afb.org

The National Association for the Deaf provides information and support for people who are hard of hearing and advocates for improved access.

National Association for the Deaf
814 Thayer Avenue
Silver Spring, MD 20910-4500
TTY: 301-587-1789
Voice: 301-587-1788
Fax: 301-587-1791
www.nad.org

The National Institute on Aging provides free information on choosing a doctor and communication with medical professionals.

National Institution on Aging
Talking to Your Doctor: A Guide for Older People
NIA Information Center
PO Box 8057
Gaithersburg, Maryland 20898-8057
www.niapublications.org

The National Family Caregivers Association seeks to support, educate and empower family caregivers and improve quality of life for caregiving families. They have a newsletter (free to caregivers) and their site has links to tips and guides on topics of interest to caregivers, such as communicating with healthcare professionals and care management techniques.

National Family Caregivers Association (NFCA)
10400 Connecticut Avenue, Suite 500
Kensington, MD 20895-3944
Tel: 301-942-6430

Toll Free: 800-896-3650
Fax: 301-942-2302
www.thefamilycaregiver.org

3

Caring for Yourself

Even if you are only starting to consider caring for a loved one in your home, you are probably aware that taking on such a responsibility would add new stress to your life. If you are already providing care, you may feel like there are times when it creates more stress than you can handle. This chapter will help you recognize the stress that is involved in caregiving and find ways to care for yourself as you care for your loved one.

First Steps

Organize and hold a family meeting involving everyone who will be participating in or making decisions about care.

Assess your own health and level of stress.

Identify ways to reduce or cope with stress in your life by developing a stress management plan.

Planning and Holding a Family Meeting

Caring for someone who is unable to care for herself is a very daunting task; it is not something that one person can do alone (Fig. 3-1). Once the decision has been made by a family that one of its members needs full-time care in the home, a family meeting should be called to make care decisions and divide the responsibilities of care. This meeting should include all family members who will be involved in any way with care and care decisions.

While every family meeting will have its own dynamic and its own questions that need to be answered, there are some general questions that should probably be addressed in some form at all initial caregiver family meetings. These include:

1. Who is the best person to be the primary caregiver? Would someone have to give up working or work less; if so, is there someone who is willing and able to do so? Do some people have homes that would work especially well, or that

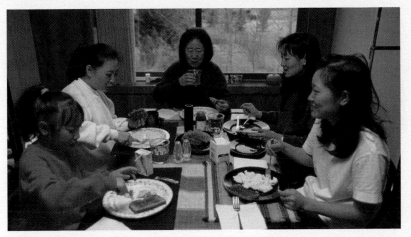

Fig. 3-1. Ideally, all family members will be involved when caring for someone who is ill or disabled.

would not work at all? How do other members of the households in question feel about becoming caregivers? Be sure to take into account the feelings of the person being cared for. Be aware that the task of primary caregiver may need to be reassigned if things do not work out due to safety or financial concerns or incompatibility issues.

2. Are there other family members who could help the primary caregiver by having the person being cared for stay with them for extended periods of time, perhaps on weekends or certain days of the month? Remember that the person being cared for does not have to stay at the same place all the time, although some sense of stability is desirable.

3. Consider the different abilities of each family member. Who has the best home environment for caregiving? The ideal home would allow quality of life for the family as well as the person being cared for, with private space available for everyone and places to entertain guests (Fig. 3-2). Who

has the most free time? Who can contribute financially? Is there someone who is a good builder who might be able to make necessary modifications to the home, or someone who is especially skilled in financial and legal matters?

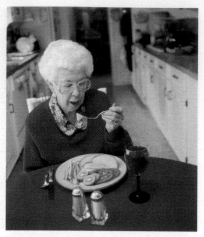

Fig. 3-2. The ideal home for caregiving should have private space as well as public space.

4. What kind of outside help can be used to fill in any gaps? Can the family afford to hire care? If not, remember that there are many sources of help that are free of charge; most of these can be found in the local telephone directory.

In order to get all of these and any other pertinent questions answered, the family meeting should be planned carefully in advance. The following are some tips for organizing a successful family meeting:

1. Try to schedule the meeting so that everyone can be in the same place at the same time. If that is not possible, those who cannot attend may be brought in via conference call.

2. Write down detailed information about the needs and limitations of the person being cared for. Include such things as modifications that would need to be made to the home of the primary caregiver, regular treatment or physician appointments that would need to be kept, and any special needs such as vision or hearing impairment, dementia or

confusion, and any illness or injury. This information should be sent out to all family members before they are asked to list their agenda items (see item #4).

3. Draft a realistic budget for all caregiving expenses and share it with family members. Remember to include such things as food, medications, adaptive devices and modifications to the home. This should also be available before the agenda is created.

4. Create an agenda. Ask each person who will attend to send in advance all items that they wish to cover. This will help ensure that nothing is missed, and the formality of the meeting format may help tone down emotions.

5. Have each participant write down and bring to the meeting a list of their skills and weaknesses and the things that he is and is not willing to do.

6. Designate a person to facilitate the meeting. This person will not be in a position of authority but rather will guide the meeting through the agenda, making sure nothing gets missed and that everyone understands the decisions that are being made. If family relations are strained or antagonistic, it might be best to get a neutral party, such as a social worker, to act in this role (Fig. 3-3).

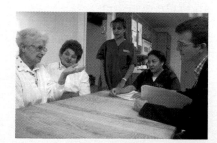

Fig. 3-3. If family relations are tense, a neutral party such as a social worker or trusted member of the care team can moderate family meetings.

7. Someone should be designated to wrap up and summarize the meeting. All decisions on all issues, especially action items, should be restated

to ensure that everyone understands and is in agreement. Someone should be assigned to write notes from the meeting and send them out to everyone within a reasonable period of time after the meeting takes place.

Family meetings do not always proceed without conflict; people may become upset and emotional and lose sight of the issues that need to be addressed. The following suggestions will help you keep the meeting running smoothly and ensure that all necessary decisions are made.

- Include the receiver of care in a dynamic role in the meeting if at all possible (Fig. 3-4). No one likes to have decisions made for her without her input, and there is a greater chance for success if the person being cared for participates in the decision-making process.

- Remember the principles of communication discussed in chapter 2. Be aware of your body language, tone of voice and facial expression, as well as those of others. Remember to be an active listener, asking for more information and repeating to make sure you have understood. Do not interrupt, and do not evade issues that make you feel uncomfortable. Use statements that focus on yourself rather than others, e.g. "I feel" instead of "you make me feel."

- Be honest and direct. If you feel that someone should be participating more or should be offer-

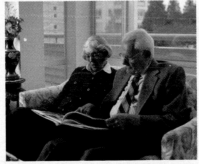

Fig. 3-4. If possible, the person being cared for should have an active role in family meetings.

ing more help than she is, ask her about it. Do not go away from the meeting with negative feelings from questions you did not ask or issues you did not address.

- Try to see the perspective of each of the other family members. If someone resists helping, find out why he is doing so before you get angry or upset. There may be things he is uncomfortable about doing, but there may be other things that he could do that he has not thought of.

- Be honest and concrete about the responsibilities that you can accept. If you are a poor organizer or uncomfortable with giving personal care, say so. Speak for yourself and do not allow other family members to choose your role for you.

- Do not allow yourself to be taken advantage of. Even if you are already designated as the primary caregiver, that does not mean that you must do everything.

- There should be a wrap-up discussion after the meeting in which all decisions are briefly restated to make sure that everyone understands what is to be done. If necessary, schedule another meeting to address any unresolved issues.

Once the caregiving responsibilities have been divided among family members, you will be able to assess your level of stress and your self-care needs.

Why is it essential to care for yourself?

You may feel that you can postpone your own needs until some later time. For example:

- After Mother is walking again, I will be able to get some exercise myself.

- When I'm no longer cooking special meals for Dad, I'll start eating better.

- After we get through this next surgery, I'll be able to take a break and have some time alone.

Certainly, in situations of serious illness it is natural to put the needs of the sick person before our own. But if we never make time for ourselves, if we never nurture ourselves, we will reach a point where we are no longer able to care for our loved ones. Ask yourself the following questions:

- Am I eating a balanced diet?

- Am I receiving preventive medical and dental care?

- Do I exercise with some regularity (Fig. 3-5)?

- Do I get a reasonable amount of sleep on a regular basis?

- Is there time in the day for me to do something for myself, such as read a book, talk to a friend, relax in front of the tele-vision, or take a walk?

- Do I get out of the house and see people outside my family?

- Do I avoid unhealthy use of alcohol and tobacco?

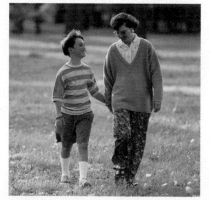

Fig. 3-5. One measurement of how well you are caring for yourself is the amount of exercise you get.

The more questions you were able to answer "yes," the better job you are doing caring for yourself even as you care for others. The more "no" answers you gave, the more your own health and well-being may be at risk.

Stress

Stress is the state of being frightened, excited, confused, in danger, or irritated. Although we usually associate stress with negative situations, positive things can cause stress, too. For example, getting married and having a baby are usually positive situations, but both can cause enormous stress due to the changes they bring to our lives (Fig 3-6).

Stress is not merely an emotional response, but a physical response. When we experience stress, changes occur in our bodies. The nervous system responds to stress by increasing heart rate, respiratory rate, and blood pressure. Thus, in a stressful situation you may notice that your heart is pounding, you are breathing hard, and you are warm or perspiring.

Each of us has a different tolerance level for stress. This level of tolerance depends on your personality and life experiences, but also on your general physical health. Re-

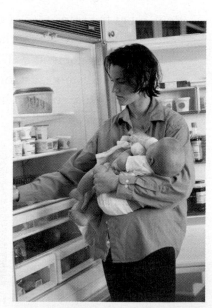

Fig. 3-6. A happy event, such as the birth of a baby, can cause stress.

search has shown that people who exercise regularly, eat a nutritious diet, and lead a healthy lifestyle are better able to handle stress. Exercise, diet, and lifestyle affect physical health, and a healthy body is more able to cope with the physical effects of stress (Fig. 3-7). In addition, exercise promotes relaxation, providing relief from the emotional effects of stress.

Various techniques can also be used to facilitate the release of stress. We can calm and relax our bodies and minds by using deep breathing, visualization, and other methods. Some of these techniques are described in this chapter. You may already have some methods that work for you. Keep in mind that stress is always present; accept that stress may be particularly intense as you care for a loved one who is ill or dying. You cannot eliminate stress from your life, but you can find ways to respond constructively, to maintain your own health and well-being, and to care for yourself as you care for others.

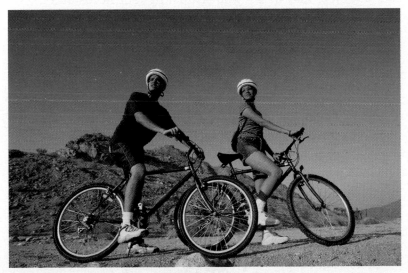

Fig. 3-7. A healthy body is better able to cope with stress.

Deep Breathing

Close your eyes and inhale through your nose as slowly and deeply as possible. Feel the air filling your lungs all the way down to your belly. When you can take in no more air, hold the breath a moment, then exhale slowly and gently through your mouth, releasing all the air and finally opening your eyes. Repeat once or twice.

Affirmations

Close your eyes and say to yourself, silently or aloud, "I am becoming more calm." Other phrases you can use include: "I am doing the best I can," "This too shall pass," "Breathe in love, breathe out fear." Using affirmations with deep breathing can be particularly effective.

Visualization: The Waterfall

Close your eyes and imagine you are under a waterfall. The force of the water is washing away your tension. Imagine the tension being washed away, one body part at a time, from your head through the soles of your feet. Visualize the tension being washed far away by the rushing water.

The Body Scan

Close your eyes. Pay attention to your breathing and posture. Be sure you are comfortable. Starting at the balls of your feet, concentrate on your feet. Discover any tension hidden in the feet. Try to relax and release the tension. Continue very slowly, taking a breath between each body part. Move up from the feet, focusing on and relaxing the legs, knees, thighs, hips, stomach, back, shoulders, neck, jaw, eyes, forehead, and scalp. Take a few very deep breaths and open your eyes.

Stress Management Plan

One of the best ways to cope with stress is to develop a plan for managing stress. The plan can include things that you will do every day as well as things to do specifically in stressful situations. When thinking about a plan, you will need to answer the following questions:

- What are the sources of stress in my life?

- When do I most often experience stress?

- What effects of stress do I see in my life?

- What can I change to decrease the stress I feel?

- What must I learn to cope with because I cannot change it?

When you have answered these questions, you will have a clearer picture of the challenges you face. Then you can try to come up with some strategies for managing stress. Write a list of things that you will do every day, such as eating breakfast and taking two or three breaks to relax and stretch. Then add in other things to do for yourself throughout the week (Fig 3-8).

A stress management plan is a great place to start to manage your stress. It will help you fit in the things that you want to do each week. You may not be able to stick to the plan exactly every week, but it will give you goals to work toward and personal time to look forward to.

Monday, Wednesday, Friday: Go for a walk after supper. Invite Chuck to go with me.

Tuesday, Saturday: Go to support group.

Sunday: Go to church. Visit friends. Plan menu for the week. Clip coupons from the paper and go grocery shopping.

Every week: Do one thing I want to do, like seeing a movie, taking a bubble bath, or reading a magazine.

Fig. 3-8.

Strategies for Coping

In addition to the above techniques for releasing stress, there are some other strategies caregivers can use to handle frustration, avoid burnout, and maintain physical and emotional health. Not all the strategies listed here will be appropriate for you, but there may be a few ideas that fit your needs and lighten the load you are carrying.

1. Give yourself credit for what you are doing. Being a caregiver is an incredibly generous, loving, and difficult role. Pat yourself on the back once in a while—or once a day!

2. Do not expect to be perfect, to get everything done, or to have everything turn out exactly the way you hoped. Remember that when you look back on this time, it will matter that you were there to provide care and support to your loved one; it will not matter that the ironing didn't get done.

3. Be positive. Think positive thoughts; seek out positive people. Avoid people who drain you of energy you need for yourself and for your loved one.

4. Set boundaries. Say "no" to activities that take more time or energy than you can spare.

5. Laugh. Watch a funny movie; read a funny book. Laughter is healing and stress-releasing (Fig. 3-9).

6. Take life one day at a time.

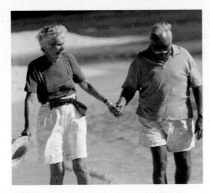

Fig. 3-9. Laughter is a great stress reliever.

7. Let others help you. Accept offers of assistance. Ask for what you need. Writing down a schedule of your loved one's appointments, treatments, medications and care may help you to more easily define what kind of help you need most. Everything does not have to be done exactly the way you would do it. It is more important for you to have a break.

8. Seek out respite care (Fig 3-10). Get out of the house. Do something you enjoy; take a walk, see a movie, get a massage, or have a chat with a friend.

9. Remember that the American Family and Medical Leave Act may allow you to take some time off from work to

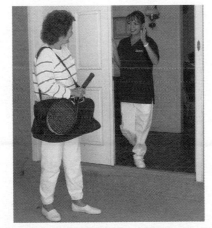

Fig. 3-10. Respite care can provide a break for caregivers.

care for your loved one at home. Check with your workplace to find out if you are eligible under this act.

10. Plan specific times to spend by yourself or with your spouse, partner, or friends (Fig. 3-11). Do not expect free time to spontaneously occur.

11. If you cannot get out, invite people over to visit. Even a talk on the phone with a friend can lift your spirits and make your day brighter.

12. Keep up with the lives and activities of your spouse, friends, and other family members as well as those of your loved one. These connections are important to your life as well.

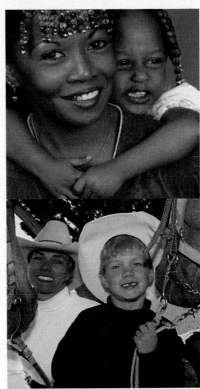

Fig. 3-11. Plan out time to spend with children and other family members.

13. Care for your body. Eat well, rest, and exercise. This will not only help you feel better, but will better enable you to do the many physically demanding tasks of caregiving. Exercise classes can be a good way to get out of the house and spend time with other people. Can your loved one exercise with you, or take classes at the same time? Many gyms offer water aerobics classes for older adults.

14. Sharing meals with friends may help you to eat better. If it is hard to get out, invite friends over for a potluck.

15. Consider joining a support group. This will give you access to information as well as support and will allow you to interact with people who can truly understand and appreciate your situation.

16. Acknowledge your feelings, whatever they may be. Express your grief, anger, frustration, fear, irritation, impatience, despair, boredom, or sadness. Write your feelings down, or talk them over with a friend or confidant or with members of your loved one's care team. Let yourself feel them. Do not judge yourself or your feelings.

Resources

Caregiver.com is an upbeat online magazine for caregivers with discussion groups and links to regional resources.

Caregiver.com
6365 Taft Street
Suite 3003
Hollywood, FL 33024
Tel: 954-893-0550
Toll-free: 800-829-2734
www.caregiver911.com

SATH provides vacation assistance for those with disabilities and advocates for better accessibility on the part of the travel and tourism industries.

Society for Accessible Travel and Hospitals (SATH)
347 Fifth Ave, Suite 610
New York, NY 10016
Tel: 212-447-7284
Fax: 212-725-8253
E-mail: sathtravel@aol.com
www.sath.org

Setting Up Your Home, Safety and Body Mechanics

Most of us live in homes that were designed, furnished and decorated for healthy, mobile occupants. When we choose to care for a loved one in a home environment, we must adapt the home to make it safe, practical, and comfortable for both the person receiving care and for those who are providing care (Fig. 4-1). This chapter will help you set up your home for caregiving with these three things in mind: safety, practicality, and comfort.

Your safety and comfort are important to consider as well. As a caregiver, you will use your body to help your loved one. You may be surprised how physically strenuous it can be. The more frail or immobile your loved one, the more you may need to help lift, transfer, and assist him in walking, standing and bathing. There are specific, correct ways that professional caregivers use their bodies in caregiving. This book will show you those ways.

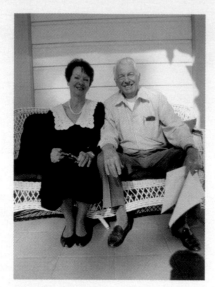

Fig. 4-1. The home should be safe, practical and comfortable for all members of the household.

First Steps

Assess and adapt your home for safety.

Assess and adapt your home for practicality, without compromising any adaptations made for safety.

Assess and adapt your home for comfort, without compromising adaptations made for safety or practicality.

Practice being aware of your body mechanics and keeping your body in alignment while standing, sitting, or lying down.

Think about the tasks you do during the day and ways to do them safely. Before starting each task, decide how best to do it with the least risk of injury.

Obtain any items that might help you do daily tasks more safely, such as step stools, gait or transfer belts for helping your loved one to stand or walk, or a hospital-type bed that could be raised to help you avoid bending.

The first step in adapting the home is to consider what you have to start with and what your needs will be. Ask yourself these questions:

- Are you moving your loved one into an unfamiliar home?

- Are there stairs? Will your loved one need to use them?

- Are there changes in the levels between rooms or are there abrupt thresholds?

- Is she suffering confusion or dementia?

- Are walkways in the home cluttered with throw rugs or with stacks of books, magazines, and papers (Figs. 4-2 and 4-3)?

- Are space heaters in use?

- Are electrical cords old, frayed, or placed where they could cause someone to trip?

- Do electrical outlets or wiring appear faulty?

- Are there smoke alarms? Do they work?

- Can a walker, wheelchair, or cane be used safely on the floor surfaces in the house?

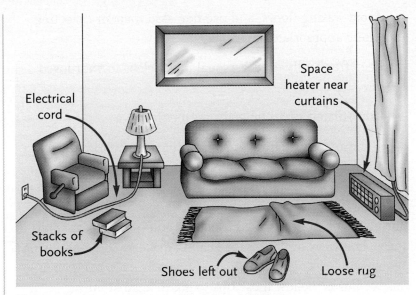

Fig. 4-2.

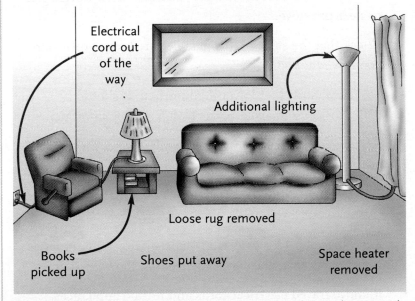

Fig. 4-3. Clutter, space heaters, and unsafe electrical cords must be removed from the home.

- Is all lighting adequate?

- Is there unnecessary furniture that could be removed and stored elsewhere?

- Does your loved one have difficulty getting in and out of bed? Up and down onto chairs or the toilet? In and out of the shower or bathtub? Note where adaptation is needed.

- Where can your loved one rest comfortably in the home? Where can he spend time comfortably with visitors or spend time reading or on hobbies?

A medical professional, such as a nurse, case manager, or occupational therapist, should be available to review and assess the home with you and your loved one.

Safety First

The first concern in adapting a home for caregiving is safety. Walk through the home looking for hazards for a person who is weak, frail, or confused. Try to anticipate potential dangers before accidents occur.

Common types of accidents that occur in the home include the following:

Falls: Falls are the leading cause of injury and related death in the home. Falls can be caused by an unsafe environment or by loss of abilities. Falls are particularly common among the elderly; one of every three persons over age 65 falls each year. According to the International Council on Active Aging, in 2002 about 12,800 persons aged 65 and older died from falls; this equals one death per hour of that year. This increased risk of falls is partly due to normal changes of aging, including slowing of reflexes, changes in depth perception, and reduced mobility. Many older adults are also taking medications that may cause them to lose their balance and fall more easily. The financial impact of these falls is significant. By 2020, the cost of fall injuries for people ages 65 and older is expected to reach $43.8 billion.

Older people are often more seriously injured by falls because their bones are more fragile; they also heal more slowly. Injury from falls is the leading cause of death for people over 65. In addition to physical injuries, people who suffer from falls can easily lose confidence in their own abilities, leading to a further loss of independence. Be especially alert for the risk of falls.

Factors that raise the risk of falls include the following:

- clutter

- throw rugs

- exposed electrical cords

- slippery floors

- uneven floors or stairs

- poor lighting

Personal conditions that raise the risk of falls include medications, loss of vision, gait or balance problems, weakness, paralysis, and disorientation.

Follow these tips to guard against falls:

- Clear all walkways of clutter, throw rugs, and cords.

- Avoid waxing floors, and use non-skid mats or carpeting where appropriate.

- Keep frequently used personal items close to your loved one.

- Immediately clean up spills on the floor.

- Mark uneven flooring or stairs with red tape to indicate a hazard.

- Improve lighting where necessary.

Burns: Burns can be caused by stoves and by electrical appliances, hot water or liquids, or heating devices. Older adults or people with loss of sensation due to paralysis are at a greater risk for burns. Follow these tips to guard against burns:

- Roll up sleeves and avoid loose clothing when working at or near the stove.

- Check that the stove and appliances are turned off when you leave the room.

- Set the water heater lower than normal. It should be set at 120°F to 130°F to avoid burns from scalding tap water.

- Always check water temperature with a water thermometer or on your wrist before using.

- Check temperatures of liquids on your wrist before serving them to your loved one.

- Keep space heaters away from beds, chairs, and draperies. Never allow space heaters to be used in the bathroom.

- Remove frayed electrical cords and unsafe appliances immediately.

Poisoning: Homes contain many harmful substances that should not be swallowed. These products should be kept in separate cabinets with childproof latches or locks. If your loved one is confused, mark these cabinets with signs that clearly indicate danger. Have the number for the Poison Control Center posted by the telephone.

Any of the following household materials can be poisonous:

- household bleach

- cleaning products (Fig. 4-4)

- aerosol or spray cans

- paint

- chemicals such as turpentine or paint thinner

- prescription and over-the-counter medicines

- hair spray

- nail polish remover

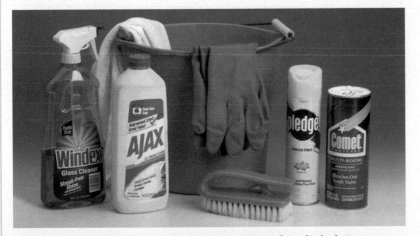

Fig. 4-4. Cleaning products can be poisonous. Keep them locked away.

If your loved one has a diminished sense of taste or smell due to stroke or head injury, she might not be able to tell when food has spoiled. Check the refrigerator and cabinets frequently for foods that are moldy, sour, or otherwise spoiled. Investigate any odors you notice. A person with dementia may hide food and let it spoil in closets, drawers, or other places.

Cuts: Cuts typically occur in the kitchen or bathroom. Keep any sharp objects, including knives, peelers, graters, food processor blades, scissors, nail clippers, or razors locked away if your loved one is confused. Know proper first aid for cuts (see chapter 13).

Choking: Choking can occur when eating, drinking, or swallowing medication. People who are weak, ill, or unconscious may choke on their own saliva. A person's tongue can also become swollen and obstruct the airway.

To guard against choking, cut food into bite-sized pieces if your loved one has trouble using utensils. He should eat in as upright a position as possible to avoid choking. If your loved one has swallowing difficulties, he may have a special diet with liquids thickened to the consistency of honey. Thickened liquids are easier to swallow (see chapter 12).

Household Tips for Preventing Accidents

Bathroom

Falls: Use non-skid bathmats in tubs and showers. Install grab bars for the tub, shower and toilet if your loved one is weak or unsteady (Figs. 4-5 and 4-6). Make sure that he is not using towel racks for support. Provide a raised toilet seat for ease of use. Provide a shower chair with non-skid feet. Make sure that all shelves are easily accessible.

Burns: Check water temperature with a bath thermometer or on your wrist. Put away electrical appliances when they are not in use. Do not use electrical appliances near a water source.

Drowning: If your loved one is ill or weak, do not leave her alone in the tub. Do not leave her alone in the tub or shower if she is dizzy or confused.

Poisoning: Store all medications in containers with childproof caps and in locked cabinets for people who are disoriented. Be sure that all medications are labeled. If your loved one has eyeglasses, make sure that he wears them when reading medication labels. Store your loved one's medications separately from

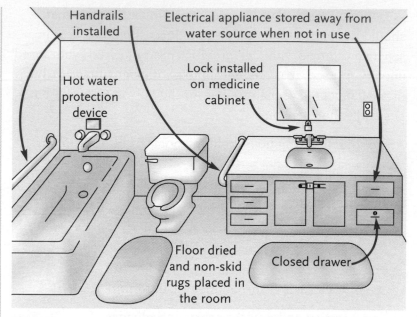

Fig. 4-6.

medications taken by other members of the household. Discard old and unused medications.

Cuts: Put away razors and other sharp objects (such as nail scissors) when they are not in use.

Kitchen

Burns: Avoid loose clothing while working in the kitchen (Figs. 4-7 and 4-8). Turn pot handles out of sight and toward the back of the stove. Stir food, especially if it has been cooked in a microwave, to ensure that it is uniformly warm and not too hot before serving. Cool hot liquids with an ice cube before serving, as appropriate. Have your loved one sit down while preparing food, if possible.

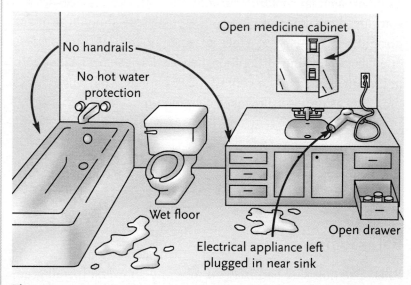

Fig. 4-5.

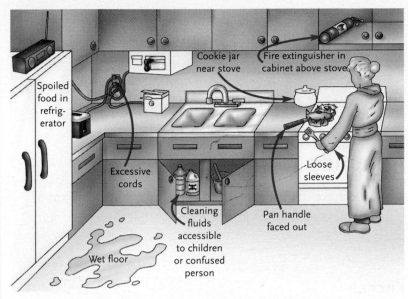

Spoiled food in refrigerator

Cookie jar near stove

Fire extinguisher in cabinet above stove

Excessive cords

Loose sleeves

Cleaning fluids accessible to children or confused person

Pan handle faced out

Wet floor

Fig. 4-7.

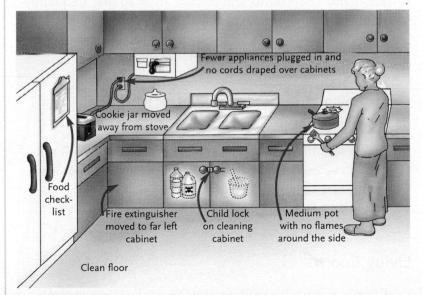

Food checklist

Cookie jar moved away from stove

Fewer appliances plugged in and no cords draped over cabinets

Fire extinguisher moved to far left cabinet

Child lock on cleaning cabinet

Medium pot with no flames around the side

Clean floor

Fig. 4-8. Prevent burns and other injuries by adapting your kitchen for safety and never wearing loose-fitting sleeves in the kitchen.

Poisoning: Keep emergency numbers, including the Poison Control Center, near the phone. Lock away all household cleaning products and other chemicals. Label storage as needed.

Cuts: Keep cutlery put away. If you are using a knife and put it down for a moment, place it away from the edge of the counter or table. Keep sharp kitchen tools in safe places.

Choking: If your loved one has difficulty swallowing, serve softer foods and foods cut into small pieces. Encourage her to take small bites of food, chew thoroughly, and eat slowly.

Bedroom

Falls: Keep a nightlight on to illuminate pathways. If your loved one has an adjustable bed, keep it in its lowest position.

Burns: Do not allow your loved one to smoke in bed or, if he is disoriented, when alone. Do not allow smoking around oxygen tanks or equipment. Place a call signal nearby so that your loved one can signal you if needed.

Cuts: Be sure sharp objects are put away.

Living Room

Falls: If your loved one needs support while walking, talk to his doctor about getting a walker or cane. If your loved one is using assistive devices for walking, make sure they are properly maintained and are being used correctly. Install handrails where necessary. Keep the floors clear. Keep electrical and extension cords out of the way. Remove low tables in pathways. Be sure that shoes are sturdy and laces are tied. Watch for pets, especially small dogs and cats.

Burns: If your loved one has dementia, keep electrical outlets covered with safety plugs. Keep lighters and matches out of sight and out of reach.

Cuts: Keep sharp objects out of reach.

Garage and Outdoors

Falls: Keep walkways clear of obstructions, snow and ice.

The following are some more general guidelines for adapting your home for safe caregiving:

- Remove or lock away all firearms and ammunition.

- Remove unnecessary furniture.

- Install handrails as needed along walls and walkways.

- Place non-skid tape on edges of stair treads.

- Clear stairs of clutter.

- Secure handrails or banisters so they are sturdy.

- Remove ill-fitting or worn slippers or shoes that could cause falls and provide shoes or slippers with non-skid soles for traction.

- Replace faulty electrical cords or outlets.

- Remove furniture that is shaky or unstable.

- Provide sturdy seating with armrests that can be used for support.

- Make sure furniture does not slide on floor surfaces.

- Keep floors clean and dry.

- If possible, use solid colors for floors as patterning (e.g. checkered, floral designs) interferes with depth perception.

- Keep room temperature in the home at least 65° F. Prolonged exposure to cold may cause a drop in body temperature, which may lead to dizziness and falling.

Adapting for Practicality

Once you have made sure the home is safe, you will want to think about making it as practical as possible. Here are some suggestions:

Kitchen

- Reorganize cupboards and storage areas so that frequently-used items are within reach.

- Leave out the one or two pans, utensils, and dishes that are most likely to be needed.

- Plan simple meals and snacks; leave all instructions and ingredients together.

- Create an eating area in the kitchen so hot food does not need to be carried to another room. Provide a sturdy chair, a clear table surface, napkins and condiments, and a telephone within reach if possible.

Living Room

- Provide a space for reading, watching television, visiting, talking on the telephone, and whatever activities your loved one can enjoy (Fig 4-9). Be sure lighting is adequate. Keep the telephone and remote controls within reach.

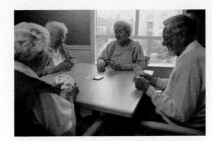

Fig. 4-9. The ideal caregiving home should have space for enjoyable activities.

- A rolling table or cart can be used to transport medications, equipment, or projects from room to room.

- Specially adapted furniture, such as a chair with a seat that mechanically rises to help a person stand, can be very helpful.

Bedroom

- If the bedroom is upstairs, consider adapting a room downstairs, even the living room, to be used as a bedroom.

- A hospital-type bed can be rented and makes care of a bedbound person much easier (Fig 4-10).

- Use a baby monitor or intercom system to communicate between rooms.

- Keep all needed supplies at the bedside: tissues, telephone, water, medica-

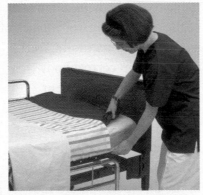

Fig. 4-10. A hospital-type bed makes care of a bedbound person much easier.

tions, a flashlight, a radio, remote control for the television, glasses, and lotion.

- A portable commode can be used in the bedroom so your loved one does not have to walk to the bathroom.

Bathroom

- Label bathroom doors if needed for someone who is disoriented.

- Have extra supplies of towels and toilet paper within reach.

- Provide a hand-held shower attachment to make bathing easier.

- Bring a cordless telephone into the bathroom.

- Be sure all necessary toiletries are within reach before beginning bathing.

Comfort in the Home

Choosing to care for someone in the home allows you to provide a wonderfully comfortable environment. A few general adaptations will help create comfortable spaces:

- Keep the temperature regulated. Age, illness, and medication can affect sensitivity to temperature. Provide extra blankets, a warm robe, and even a soft wool cap indoors. Consider a heat lamp in the bathroom.

- Although it is important to reduce clutter for safety, try to retain the homelike feeling of the house. Be sure family photos or other memorabilia are displayed. For a bedbound person, place some pleasant things to look at within view.

A fish tank can be very entertaining.

- Create a space where visitors can be welcomed without invading the comfort or privacy of the home (Fig 4-11). Have extra chairs that can be brought out for visitors and then put out of the way when they leave.

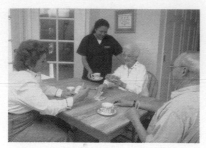

Fig. 4-11. Space should be created in the home for entertaining visitors.

The extent to which you adapt your home for caregiving will depend on your budget, the needs of your loved one, and the home itself. Use the suggestions above as a starting point in making the necessary adaptations to create a safe, practical, and comfortable environment. Remember that many resources are available to help in adapting the home. As always, check with your Area Agency on Aging, as well as the many websites and newsletters for family caregivers. Hospital and healthcare supply stores will also have many adaptive devices for rent or purchase.

Body Mechanics

Back strain or injury is one of the greatest risks of working in the home. Prevention is very important. In this book we will illustrate the correct procedures for helping your loved one stand, change positions, and walk. These procedures will include instructions for maintaining proper body mechanics.

Body mechanics is the way the parts of the body work together as you move. When used properly, good body mechanics can save energy and prevent injury by enabling you to effectively push, pull, and lift objects as well as people who are not able to fully support or move their own bodies. Understanding some basic principles will help you develop proper body mechanics.

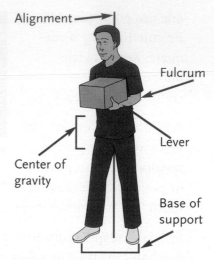

Fig. 4-12. Proper body alignment is achieved when a straight line can be drawn through the body's center of gravity.

Alignment: The concept of alignment is based on the word "line." When you stand up straight, a vertical line can be drawn right through the center of your body and your center of gravity. When the line is straight, the body is in alignment (Fig. 4-12). A body does not have to be standing up to be in alignment; when sitting or lying down, you should also try to have your body in alignment. This means that the two sides of the body are mirror images of each other, with the body parts lined up naturally. You can maintain correct body alignment when lifting or carrying an object by keeping the object close to your body and in front of you (Fig. 4-13). Point your feet and body in the direction you are moving. Avoid twisting at the waist.

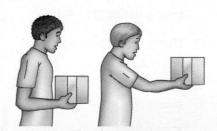

Fig. 4-13. Hold objects close to your body when carrying them. The person on the right is more likely to strain his muscles.

Base of support: The base of support is the foundation that supports an object. Something that has a wide base of support is more stable than something with a narrow base of support. For example, a tricycle is much harder to tip over than a bicycle or a unicycle. This is also true for the human body. The feet are the body's base of support. A person who is standing with legs apart has a greater base of support, and so is more stable, than someone standing with his feet close together.

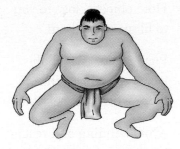

Fig. 4-14. A low center of gravity gives a more stable base of support.

Center of gravity: The center of gravity in your body is the point where the most weight is concentrated. This point will depend on the position the body is in. When you stand, your weight is centered in your pelvis. A low center of gravity gives a more stable base of support (Fig. 4-14). Putting heavy books on the top of a narrow bookshelf will make the shelf top-heavy and more likely to tip over. Putting heavy books on the bottom shelf and lighter books above them lowers the center of gravity, making the bookshelf more stable. Bending your knees when lifting an object lowers your pelvis and, therefore, lowers your center of gravity. This gives you more stability and makes you less likely to fall or strain your working muscles.

Fulcrum and lever: A lever moves an object by resting on a base of support, called a fulcrum. Think of a seesaw on a playground. The flat board you sit on is the lever. The triangular base the board rests on is the fulcrum. When two children sit on opposite sides of the seesaw, they easily move each other up

and down. They can do this because the fulcrum and lever of the seesaw are actually doing the work.

If you think of your body as a set of fulcrums and levers, you can find smart ways to lift without working as hard. Think of your arm as a lever with the elbow as its fulcrum. When you lift something, resting it against your forearm will shorten the lever and make it easier to lift than holding it in your hands.

By applying the principles of body mechanics to your daily activities, you can avoid injury and use less energy to accomplish your duties. Some common examples of applying body mechanics include the following:

Lifting a heavy object from the floor. To lift a heavy object from the floor, spread your feet shoulder-width apart and bend your knees. Using the strong, large muscles in your thighs, upper arms, and shoulders, lift the object. Pull it close to your body to a point level with your pelvis. By doing this you are keeping the object close to your center of gravity and base of support. When you stand up, push with your strong hip and thigh muscles to raise your body and the object together (Fig. 4-15).

Do not twist when you are moving an object. Always face the object or person you are moving. Pivot your feet instead of twisting at the waist.

Helping your loved one sit up, stand up, or walk. When you need to support a person's weight, protect yourself by assuming a good stance. Place your feet about 12 inches, or hip-width apart,

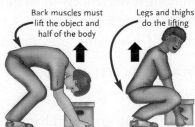

Fig. 4-15. Which of these people is lifting correctly?

one foot in front of the other, with knees bent. Your upper body should stay upright and in alignment. In this good stance, you give yourself a wide base of support and a low center of gravity. If the person starts to fall, you will be in a good position to help support her. Never try to "catch" someone who is falling. If the person falls, assist him or her to the floor. If you try to reverse a fall in progress, you are likely to injure yourself or the other person (Fig. 4-16).

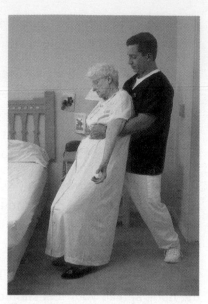

Fig. 4-16. Never try to catch someone who is falling; instead support her and ease her to the floor.

Bend your knees to lower yourself, rather than bending from the waist. When a task requires bending, use a good stance. This allows you to use the big muscles in your legs and hips rather than straining the smaller muscles in your back.

If you are making an adjustable bed, adjust the height to a safe working level, usually waist high. If you are making a regular bed, put one knee on the bed, lean, or even kneel to support yourself at working level. Avoid bending at the waist.

In addition, keep the following tips in mind to avoid strain and injury:

- Use both arms and hands when lifting, pulling, pushing, or carrying objects.

- Hold objects close to you to lift or carry them.

- Push, slide, or pull objects rather than lifting them whenever possible.

- Avoid bending and reaching as much as possible (Fig 4-17). Move or position furniture so that you do not have to bend or reach.

- Avoid twisting at the waist. Instead, turn your whole body. Your feet should point toward the object you are lifting.

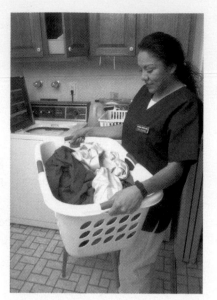

Fig. 4-17. Avoid reaching or bending. For example, put the clothes basket on a chair before putting clothes into it.

- Get help whenever possible for lifting or assisting your loved one.

- Let your loved one know what you will do so he can help if possible. Count to three and lift or move on three so that everyone moves together. Never attempt to lift an object or a person that you feel you cannot handle.

The following are several strategies that can help you apply good body mechanics in the home:

Have the right tools for a job. For example, if you cannot reach an object on a high shelf, use a step stool rather than climbing on a counter or straining to reach.

Have footrests and pillows available. You can make any position safer and more comfortable by using footrests and pillows to keep the body in alignment. For example, tasks that require standing for long periods can be more comfortable if you rest one foot on a footrest. This position flexes the muscles in the lower back and keeps the spine in alignment. When sitting, using a footrest allows for a more comfortable leg position. Crossing the legs disrupts alignment and should be avoided. Using pillows can make any chair more comfortable. Use pillows behind the back or in the small of the back to keep the back straight.

Keep tools, supplies, and clutter off the floor. Keep frequently-used items on shelves or counters where they can be easily reached without stretching. Keeping things organized will also help you find what you need without straining.

Sit when you can. Whenever you can sit to do a job, do so. Chopping vegetables, folding clothes, and many other tasks can be done easily while sitting. For jobs like scouring the bathtub, kneel or use a low stool. Avoid bending at the waist.

There are devices called "gait" and "transfer" belts that can help you when you are moving your loved one or helping him to walk (Fig. 4-18). In chapter 10 we will describe and illustrate the correct procedures for safely assisting someone to move and walk.

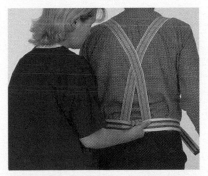

Fig. 4-18. A gait belt or transfer belt can assist you when moving a person or helping him to walk.

Resources

The Center for Healthy Aging has launched a new fall prevention action plan. The site contains statistics, information on fall prevention, and tips for modifying the home to prevent falls.

Center for Healthy Aging
300 D Street, SW, Ste. 801
Washington, D.C. 20024
Tel: 202-479-1200
Fax: 202-479-0735
TDD: 202-479-6674
www.healthyagingprograms.org

This site contains information on avoiding back injury and about conditions that can cause back pain and treatment for them.

SpineUniverse.com
1737 S. Naperville Rd. Suite 203
Wheaton, IL, 60187
www.spineuniverse.com

This website from the University of Southern California contains articles about home modification and links concerning home modification and other aging issues.

National Resource Center on Supportive Housing and Home Modification
Andrus Gerontology Center, University of Southern California
3715 McClintock Avenue
Los Angeles, CA 90089-0191
Tel: 213-740-1364
Fax: 213-740-7069

Email: homemods@usc.edu
www.homemods.org

This website has a comprehensive section on home modification, including information on where to get help for people who cannot do the modifications themselves. A form for e-mail questions and comments is provided on the website.

CarePathways.com
Tel: 1-877-521-9987
www.carepathways.com

The NAHB Research Center was created by the National Association of Home Builders to facilitate liaisons between builders, government, and industry to advance housing technology and make housing more affordable. The site has a section dedicated to senior housing which contains information about home modification for accessibility and assistive devices for the home. There are also links to checklists for interior and exterior modifications to the home and an online bookstore.

National Association of Home Builders Research Center (NAHB)
400 Prince George's Boulevard
Upper Marlboro, Maryland 20774
Telephone: 301-249-4000
Toll-free 800-638-8556
Fax: 301-430-6180
www.nahbrc.org

Preventing Infection in the Home

Aging, illness, and frailty cause people to become more susceptible to infection. The elderly are at a higher risk for infection due, in part, to weakened immune systems as a result of aging. Weakened immune systems can also result from chronic illnesses. Other factors that increase this risk are decreased circulation, slow wound healing, and malnutrition. Lack of mobility increases the risk of pressure sores, which may become infected. More frequent hospitalization makes older adults more likely to get infections. Difficulty swallowing and incontinence increase the risk of respiratory and urinary tract infections. Some medications, catheters, and other types of tubes also increase the risk of infection.

Whether your loved one is a frail, elderly person, has a immune system suppressed by chemotherapy, or is living with an infectious disease like hepatitis, you must try to prevent the spread of infection in the home. Infection is more dangerous for the elderly; even a simple cold can turn into a life-threatening illness such as pneumonia. It also may take longer for older people to recover from infection or illness. This is why preventing infection is so important. This chapter explains the causes of infection and describes measures to control and reduce the spread of infection in the home.

First Steps

Consult with your loved one's physician to find out what kind of personal protective equipment (PPE—see later in the chapter for more information) you will need to wear while caring for your loved one and when it will need to be worn. Consult with the doctor again if conditions change or if your loved one or someone else in the home develops an infectious disease.

Make sure all needed PPE and cleaning supplies are available in the home, including biohazard containers and other supplies needed to clean and dispose of waste containing body fluids.

Remember that you do not have to do everything by yourself; if you need help with the demanding task of maintaining a clean environment in your home, you can ask for or hire someone to help you.

In health care, "infection control" is the set of methods used to control and prevent the spread of disease. Infections occur

when harmful microorganisms, called pathogens, enter the body. The term "asepsis" describes a state in which no pathogens are present. It refers to the clean conditions you want to create in the home. To better understand how to prevent disease, you must first understand how it is spread.

The chain of infection describes how disease is transmitted from one being to another (Fig. 5-1). Definitions and examples of the six links in the chain of infection are:

Link 1: The causative agent is a pathogen or microorganism that causes disease. Normal flora are the microorganisms that live in the body. They do not cause harm. When they enter a different part of the body, they may cause an infection. Causative agents include bacteria, viruses, fungi, and protozoa.

Link 2: A reservoir is where the pathogen lives and grows. It can be a person, animal, plant, soil or substance. Microorganisms grow best in warm, dark, and moist places where food is present. Some microorganisms need oxygen to survive; others

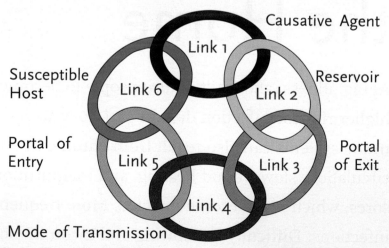

Fig. 5-1. The chain of infection shows how infection is transmitted.

do not. Reservoirs include the lungs, blood, and large intestine.

Link 3: The portal of exit is any opening on an infected person allowing pathogens to leave (Fig. 5-2). These include the nose, mouth, eyes, or a cut in the skin.

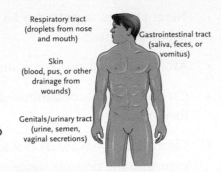

Respiratory tract (droplets from nose and mouth)

Gastrointestinal tract (saliva, feces, or vomitus)

Skin (blood, pus, or other drainage from wounds)

Genitals/urinary tract (urine, semen, vaginal secretions)

Fig. 5-2. Portals of exit allow infection to leave the body.

Link 4: The mode of transmission describes how the pathogen travels from one person to another. Transmission can happen through the air. It can also occur through direct or indirect contact. Direct contact happens by touching the infected person or his secretions. Indirect contact results from touching something contaminated by the infected person, such as a tissue or clothes.

Link 5: The portal of entry is any body opening on an uninfected person that lets pathogens enter (Fig. 5-3). These include the nose, mouth, eyes, other mucous membranes, a cut in the skin, or dry or cracked skin. Mucous membranes include the linings of the mouth, nose, eyes, rectum, or genitals.

Link 6: A susceptible host is an uninfected person who could get sick.

If one of the links of the chain of infection is broken,

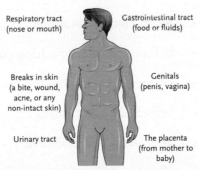

Respiratory tract (nose or mouth)

Gastrointestinal tract (food or fluids)

Breaks in skin (a bite, wound, acne, or any non-intact skin)

Genitals (penis, vagina)

Urinary tract

The placenta (from mother to baby)

Fig. 5-3. A portal of entry is a body opening on an uninfected person through which pathogens may enter.

then the spread of infection stops. Infection control practices help stop pathogens from traveling (Link 4) and getting on the hands, nose, eyes, mouth, skin, etc. (Link 5). You can also reduce your own chances of getting sick by having immunizations (Link 6) for diseases such as hepatitis B and influenza.

Standard Precautions

Standard Precautions is a method of infection control defined by the Centers for Disease Control and Prevention (CDC), a government agency. Under state and federal laws, healthcare providers are required to follow certain precautions when caring for people. Although the purpose of this book is to educate non-professional caregivers, the next few pages will include information very similar to what is used in training paid caregivers. Knowing Standard Precautions will help you understand the guidelines that the professionals providing care to your loved one are required to follow.

Following Standard Precautions means treating all blood, body fluids, non-intact skin (like abrasions, pimples, or open sores), and mucous membranes (linings of mouth, nose, eyes, rectum, penis or vagina) as if they were infected with a contagious disease. Standard Precautions include the measures listed below:

- Wear gloves if you may come into contact with blood, body fluids or secretions, broken skin (including abrasions, acne, cuts, stitches, and staples), or mucous membranes. Such situations include mouth care; bathroom assistance; care of the area around, between and including the genitals; assistance with a bedpan or urinal; ostomy care; cleaning up spills; cleansing basins, urinals, bedpans, and other containers that have held body fluids; and disposing of wastes.

- Wash your hands before putting on gloves and immediately after removing your gloves.

- Remove your gloves immediately when finished with a procedure.

- Immediately wash all skin surfaces that have been contaminated with blood and body fluids.

- Wear a disposable gown if you may come into contact with blood or body fluids (for example, when emptying a urinary drainage bag).

- Wear a mask and protective goggles if you may come into contact with splashing or spraying blood or body fluids (for example, when emptying a bedpan).

- Wear gloves and use caution when handling razor blades, needles, and other sharp objects. Discard these objects carefully in a puncture-resistant biohazard container (Fig. 5-4).

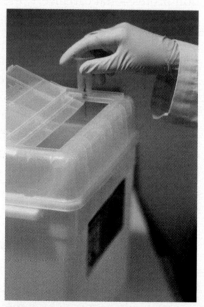

Fig. 5-4. Dispose of syringes and other sharp objects in a biohazard container.

- Never attempt to put a cap on a needle. Dispose of it in an approved container.

- Avoid nicks and cuts when shaving someone.

- Carefully bag all contaminated supplies and dispose of them properly.

- Clearly label body fluids that are being saved for a specimen with the person's name and a biohazard label. Keep them in a container with a lid.

- Dispose of contaminated wastes properly.

- Waste containing blood or body fluids is considered biohazardous waste and should be disposed of separately from household garbage.

Transmission of most infectious diseases can be prevented by always taking a few simple precautions. Washing your hands is the most important thing you can do to greatly reduce the spread of infection. All caregivers and visitors should wash their hands frequently.

You should wash your hands:

- when arriving at home

- before and after touching your loved one

- before and after making meals or working in the kitchen

- before and after eating

- after using the restroom

- after touching any item used by or for your loved one

- after smoking

- after blowing your nose, coughing or sneezing into your hand

- after touching garbage or trash

- before leaving the home

- before touching clean supplies or medications

- after removing gloves or any type of personal protection equipment (PPE), such as a protective gown or mask

- after touching a surface that may be contaminated with any body fluid

The procedure for handwashing below is the first of many procedures described in this book. In some procedures, such as those in which you may come into contact with body fluids, you will always need to wear gloves. This instruction will be included as part of the procedure. For all other procedures, you will need to wear gloves if there is broken skin on your hands or on any parts of your loved one's body that you will be touching, even though it is not included as part of the procedure.

Washing hands

Equipment: bar or liquid soap, paper towels

1　Turn on water at sink. Keep your clothes dry; moisture breeds bacteria.

2　Angle your arms down, holding your hands lower than your elbows. This prevents water from running up your arm. Wet hands and wrists thoroughly (Fig. 5-5).

3　Use a generous amount of soap. Rub hands together and fingers between each other to create a lather. Lather all surfaces of fingers and hands, including above the wrists, producing friction for at least 10 seconds. Friction helps clean (Fig. 5-6).

4　Clean your nails by pushing soap under your fingernails and cuticles with a brush or by rubbing them in the palm of your hand (Fig. 5-7).

5　Being careful not to touch the sink, rinse thoroughly under running water. Rinse from just above the wrists down to your fingertips. Do not run water over unwashed arms down to clean hands (Fig. 5-8).

6　Use a clean paper towel to dry from tips of fingers up to clean wrists. Again, do not wipe towel on unwashed forearms and then wipe clean hands. Dispose of the towel without touching the waste container. If your

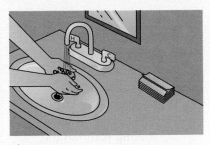

Fig. 5-5.

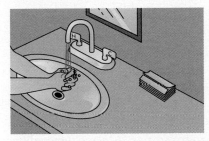

Fig. 5-6.

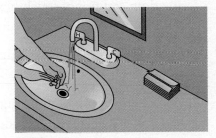

Fig. 5-7.

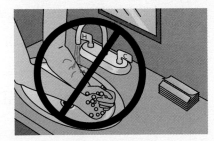

Fig. 5-8.

hands ever touch the sink or waste container, start over.

7   Use a clean, dry paper towel to turn off the faucet without contaminating your hands (Fig. 5-9). Properly discard the towel.

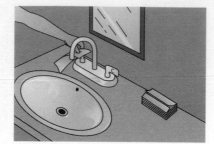

Fig. 5-9.

Gloves

You should wear gloves when there is a chance you might come into contact with body fluids, open wounds, or mucous membranes. Always wear gloves for the following tasks:

* any time you might touch blood or any body fluid, including vomit, urine, feces or saliva

* when performing or assisting with mouth care or care of any mucous membrane

* when performing or assisting with care of the perineal area (the area between and including the anus and the genitals)

* when performing care when your loved one's skin is broken by abrasions, cuts, rash, acne, pimples, or boils

* when you have open sores or cuts on your hands

* when shaving your loved one

* when disposing of soiled bed linens, gowns, dressings, and pads

If you have cuts or sores on your hands, first cover these areas

with bandages or gauze, and then put on gloves. Disposable gloves are worn only once; they should not be washed or disinfected for reuse. Replace disposable gloves as soon as they are torn. Wash your hands before putting on fresh gloves. Some people are allergic to the latex used in some gloves. If you notice a reaction, discontinue using latex gloves and look for a non-allergenic type at a medical supply store.

Putting on gloves

1	Wash your hands.
2	If you are right-handed, remove one glove from the box and slide it onto your left hand (reverse if left-handed).
3	Pulling out another glove with your gloved hand, slide your other hand into the second glove.
4	Interlace fingers to smooth out folds and create a comfortable fit.
5	Carefully look for tears, holes, or discolored spots; replace the glove if necessary.
6	If wearing a gown, pull the cuff of the gloves over the sleeve of the gown (Fig. 5-10).

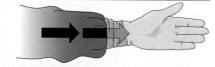

Fig. 5-10.

Remember, you are wearing gloves to protect your skin from becoming contaminated. After a procedure, your gloves are contaminated. If you open a door with your gloved hand, the doorknob becomes contaminated. Later, when you open the door with an ungloved hand, you will be infected even though you wore gloves during the procedure. It is a common mistake, after carefully putting on PPE, to contaminate the room around you. Don't do this. Before touching surfaces, remove your gloves. Wash your hands, and put on new gloves if necessary.

Taking off gloves

1	Touching only the outside of one glove, pull the first glove off by pulling down from the cuff (Fig. 5-11).
2	As the glove comes off your hand, it should be turned inside out.

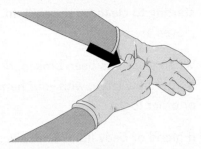

Fig. 5-11.

3	With the fingertips of your gloved hand, hold the glove you just removed. With your ungloved hand, reach two fingers inside the remaining glove, being careful not to touch any part of the outside (Fig. 5-12).

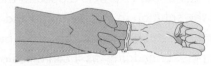

Fig. 5-12.

4	Pull down, turning this glove inside out and over the first glove as you remove it.
5	You should be holding one glove from its clean inner side; the other glove should be inside it.
6	Drop both gloves into the proper container.
7	Wash your hands.

In the medical profession, protective gowns, masks, and goggles, along with gloves, are called "personal protective equipment," or PPE. The guidelines for wearing PPE are the same as for gloves. You should wear PPE if there is a chance you could come into contact with body fluids, mucous membranes, or open wounds. Masks and goggles are worn when splashing of body fluids or blood could occur. Masks should also be worn if your loved one has a respiratory illness. This might mean you will wear PPE all the time. Speak with the doctor or nurse about when gowns, masks, and eye protection are appropriate (Fig. 5-13).

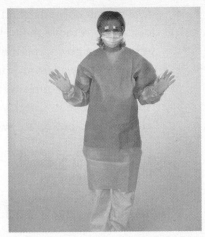

Fig. 5-13. PPE should be worn if there is any chance of contact with body fluids.

Putting on a gown

1	Wash your hands.
2	Open the gown. Hold the gown out in front of you and allow it to open (Fig. 5-14). Do not shake it. Slip your arms into the sleeves and pull the gown on.
3	Tie the neck ties into a bow so they can be easily untied later.
4	Reaching behind you, pull the gown until it completely covers your clothes. Tie the back ties (Fig. 5-15).

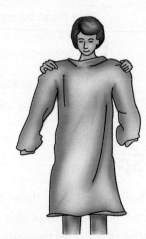

Fig. 5-14.

5 Use gowns only once and then discard or remove them. When removing a gown, roll the dirty side in and away from your body. If your gown becomes wet or soiled, remove it. Check your clothing and put on a new gown.

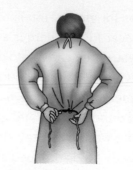

6 Put on gloves after putting on a gown.

Fig. 5-15.

Putting on a mask and goggles

1 Wash your hands.

2 Pick up the mask by the top strings or the elastic strap. Be careful not to touch the mask where it will touch your face.

3 Adjust the mask over your nose and mouth. Tie the top strings first, then the bottom strings. Masks must always be dry or they must be replaced. Never wear a mask hanging from only the bottom ties (Fig. 5-16).

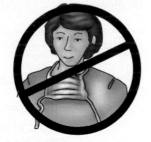

4 Put on the goggles.

Fig. 5-16.

5 Put on gloves after putting on mask and goggles.

Spills

Spills, especially those involving blood, body fluids, or glass, can pose a serious risk of infection. Using the right equipment and procedure to clean spills can eliminate this risk.

Cleaning Spills Involving Blood, Body fluids, or Glass

When blood or body fluids are spilled, put on gloves before starting to clean up the spill. In some cases, industrial strength gloves are best.

When glass has been broken, do not pick up any pieces, no matter how large, with your hands. Use a dustpan and broom or other tools.

If blood or body fluids are spilled on a hard surface such as a linoleum floor or countertop, clean it immediately using a solution of one part household bleach to ten parts water. Mix the solution in a bucket and, with gloves on, wipe up the spill with rags or paper towels dipped in the solution. You can also mix the solution in a spray bottle and spray the spill before wiping. Be careful not to spill bleach or bleach solution on clothes, carpets, or bedding, as it can discolor and damage fabrics.

If blood or body fluids are spilled on fabrics such as carpets, bedding, or clothes, do not use bleach to clean the spill. Commercial disinfectants that do not contain bleach are available. If you have no disinfectant, wear gloves and wipe spills using soap and water. Then clean carpet with regular carpet cleaner. Wear gloves while loading soiled bedding or clothes into the washing machine and add color-safe bleach to the washer with the laundry detergent.

Waste containing broken glass, blood, or body fluids should be properly bagged. Put the waste in one trash bag and close it properly. Then put the first bag inside a second, clean trash bag and close it. This is called "double-bagging." Waste containing blood or body fluids may need to be placed in a special biohazard waste bag and disposed of separately from household trash. These special bags may be provided to you or purchased from a medical supply store.

Infectious Diseases

Microorganisms carried in the blood transmit bloodborne diseases. These microorganisms may also be present in body fluids, non-intact skin (such as open sores or acne), and mucous membranes.

Bloodborne diseases can be transmitted if infected blood enters the bloodstream or if infected semen or vaginal secretions contact the mucous membranes. A person can become infected with a bloodborne disease by having sexual contact with someone carrying that disease. It is not necessary to have sexual intercourse to transmit disease. Other kinds of sexual activity can just as easily cause infection. Using a needle to inject drugs and sharing needles with others can also transmit bloodborne diseases. In addition, infected mothers may transmit bloodborne diseases to their babies in the womb or during birth.

When caring for a person with an infectious bloodborne disease, follow the doctor's instructions carefully. They will generally include the following guidelines:

- Always follow Standard Precautions.

- Wash your hands frequently, especially after personal care.

- Use PPE when needed.

- Follow isolation procedures if recommended.

- Handle laundry, personal items, and waste carefully.

Remember that you can safely touch, hug, and spend time with a loved one who has a bloodborne disease. She needs thoughtful, personal attention. Follow Standard Precautions to protect yourself, but never isolate someone emotionally because she has an infectious disease.

Sometimes the doctor will order isolation precautions. These are also known as "Transmission-Based Precautions." When infectious disease is present, special isolation precautions are required to keep the infection isolated, or separate from uninfected members of the household, including you. It is for your safety and the safety of others in the home that these precautions must be followed.

There are three categories of isolation precautions. The type used depends on the disease and how it spreads to others. They may also be used in combination for diseases that have multiple routes of transmission. **Isolation precautions are always used in addition to Standard Precautions.** Below are the isolation categories, the diseases they are intended to isolate, and some of the precautions that are appropriate.

Airborne Precautions are used for diseases that can be transmitted or spread through the air after being expelled by an infected person. The pathogens are so small that they can attach to moisture in the air and remain floating for some time (Fig. 5-17). For certain care procedures you may be required to wear a special mask to avoid being infected. Airborne diseases include tuberculosis, measles, and chicken pox. A section on tuberculosis is found later in this chapter.

Droplet Precautions are used when the disease-causing microorganism does not stay suspended in the air and usually travels only short distances after being expelled (Fig. 5-18). Droplets can be generated by coughing, sneezing, talking, or laughing. Droplet Precautions can include wearing a face mask during care procedures and restricting visits from uninfected people. Cover your nose and mouth with a tissue when you sneeze or cough and ask others to do the same. If you sneeze on your hands, wash them promptly.

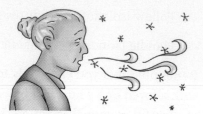

Fig. 5-17. Airborne diseases remain floating in the air for some time.

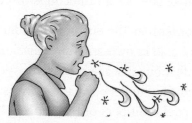

Fig. 5-18. Droplet precautions are used for microorganisms that travel only a short distance after being expelled.

Contact Precautions are used when a person is at risk of transmitting or contracting a microorganism from touching an infected object or person (Fig. 5-19). For example, bacteria could infect an open skin wound. Lice, scabies (a skin disease that causes itching), and conjunctivitis (pink eye) are examples. Transmission can occur with skin-to-skin contact during transfers or bathing. Precautions include personal protective equipment and isolation. Contact

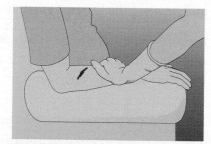

Fig. 5-19. Contact precautions are used for diseases that may be transmitted by touch.

Precautions require washing hands with antimicrobial soap and not touching infected surfaces with ungloved hands or uninfected surfaces with contaminated gloves.

Always remember that it is the disease, not the person, that is being isolated. Talk about why these special steps are being taken so that feelings are not hurt.

GUIDELINES

Isolation Procedures

Serve food using disposable dishes and utensils that are discarded in specially marked bags and stored in covered garbage containers. When these items cannot be discarded, they must be washed thoroughly in very hot water with detergent and bleach. Uninfected family members should use separate dishes and utensils.

Wear disposable gloves when handling soiled laundry. Bag laundry in the infected person's room and carry it to the laundry area in the bag. Wash this laundry separately using hot water and detergent.

A solution of bleach and water (1:10) should be mixed in a clearly labeled plastic spray bottle and stored in a safe place. The bleach solution can be used to clean up spills of blood or body fluids and to disinfect surfaces that may have been contaminated.

A person in contact or airborne isolation should use a separate bathroom. If he uses the same bathroom as other family members, it must be disinfected after each use.

Remember that these isolation precautions are always used in addition to the Standard Precautions described earlier.

In the healthcare setting, contact with infected blood or body fluids is the most common way to be infected with a bloodborne disease. Standard Precautions, handwashing, isolation, and using gloves, masks, gowns, and eye protection are all methods of preventing transmission of bloodborne diseases.

HIV and Hepatitis Infection

The major bloodborne diseases in the United States are acquired immune deficiency syndrome (AIDS) and hepatitis. HIV is the virus that causes AIDS. HIV stands for human immunodeficiency virus. HIV weakens the immune system so that the body cannot effectively fight infections. Some people with HIV will develop AIDS as a result of their HIV infection. People with AIDS lose all ability to fight infection and can die from illnesses that a healthy body could fight.

Depending on the community, many resources and services may be available for people with HIV/AIDS. These may include counseling, meal services, access to experimental drugs and any number of other services. Look in the phone book or on the Internet for resources available in your area. A social worker or another member of the care team may be able to coordinate services for people with HIV/AIDS.

Hepatitis is an inflammation of the liver caused by infection. Liver function can be permanently damaged by hepatitis, which can lead to other chronic, life-long illnesses. Several different viruses can cause hepatitis; the most common are hepatitis A, B, and C. Hepatitis B and C are bloodborne diseases that can cause death. Many more people have hepatitis B (HBV) than HIV. The risk of acquiring hepatitis is greater than the risk of acquiring HIV. The HBV vaccine can help prevent hepatitis B. There is no vaccine for hepatitis C.

Tuberculosis

Tuberculosis, or TB, is an airborne disease carried on mucous droplets suspended in the air. When a person infected with TB talks, coughs, breathes, or sings, he or she may release mucous droplets carrying the disease. TB usually infects the lungs, causing coughing, difficulty breathing, fever, and fatigue. If left untreated, TB may cause death.

There are two types of TB: 1) TB infection, also called latent TB, and 2) TB disease, also called active TB. Someone with TB infection carries the disease but does not show symptoms and cannot infect others. A person with active TB, or TB disease, shows symptoms of the disease and can spread TB to others. TB infection can progress to TB disease.

TB is more likely to be spread in small, confined, or poorly ventilated places. TB disease is more likely to develop in people whose immune systems are weakened by illness, malnutrition, alcoholism or drug abuse. People with cancer and people with HIV/AIDS are especially susceptible to developing TB disease when exposed. This is due to their weakened immune systems.

GUIDELINES
Tuberculosis

Follow Standard Precautions and Airborne Precautions.

Wear a mask and gown during care. Special masks, such as N95 or high efficiency particulate air (HEPA) masks, may be needed (Fig. 5-20). These masks filter out very small particles, such as the germs that cause TB.

Use special care when handling sputum or phlegm.

Ensure proper ventilation in the home. Open windows when possible.

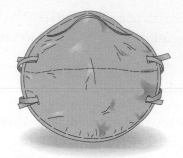

Fig. 5-20. A N95 respirator may be used to prevent the spread of TB.

Follow isolation procedures for airborne diseases if indicated.

Help your loved one remember to take all medication prescribed. Failure to take all medication is a major factor in the spread of TB.

Maintaining a Clean and Healthy Home

The rest of this chapter discusses the housekeeping tasks required when caring for someone in the home. Special attention is given to handling body wastes, as many caregivers are living with a loved one who is incontinent.

GUIDELINES
Housekeeping

Maintain a safe environment as well as a clean and healthy one. Do not wax floors if your loved one is unsteady. Clean up spills immediately (Fig. 5-21). Do not leave cleaning equipment around.

Use housekeeping procedures and methods that promote good health. Many diseases may be transmitted through improper food handling, dishwashing, handwashing, and unclean bathrooms and kitchens.

Use good body mechanics while performing home maintenance activities to prevent injury and reduce fatigue. Review the principles of body mechanics in chapter 4. Housecleaning can require a great deal of bending, standing, stooping, and lifting. Be aware of your posture. Kneel instead of stooping for long periods.

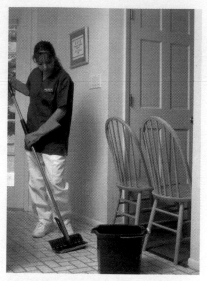

Fig. 5-21. Mop up spills quickly if your loved one is unsteady.

A clean, organized, and odor-free bathroom is an important part of improving a family's hygiene and safety (Fig. 5-22). Because it is moist and warm, the bathroom is a reservoir for the growth of microorganisms, mold, and mildew. It is a good idea to wear gloves when cleaning a bathroom.

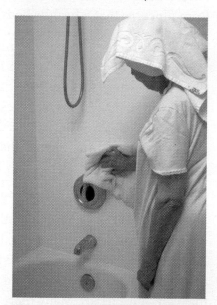

Fig. 5-22. All surfaces in the bathroom should be thoroughly cleaned.

Use a separate sponge for each area of the bathroom; use one for surfaces, another for the toilet, and a third for the shower and tub. Start with the cleanest surface first, then move to dirtier areas. Be careful not to mix different cleaners as a dangerous chemical reaction could occur. After cleaning the floor, dry it carefully to avoid accidents.

GUIDELINES

Handling Body Wastes and Incontinence

Wear gloves and a gown when handling bedpans, urinals, incontinence pads, dressings, or anything that contains or has contacted body wastes (urine, feces, blood, vomit, phlegm or mucus). Urine irritates the skin and should be washed off completely after any occurrence of incontinence.

Flush the contents of urinals and bedpans down the toilet. Incontinence pads or garments and dressings should be sealed in a plastic bag, put in another plastic bag and sealed before removal from the person's room or bathroom.

If your loved one has a bloodborne infection, you should have special biohazardous waste bags to use for waste disposal.

Clothing, bed sheets and other non-disposable items that contact body waste should be soaked in a bucket in a solution of hot water, detergent, and household disinfectant. They can then be washed in the washing machine in hot water and detergent.

Hard surfaces that contact body wastes can be cleaned with paper towels and bleach or bleach solution from a spray bottle. Wear gloves while performing these clean-ups.

Always remove and dispose of gloves properly after each use;
never attempt to disinfect or reuse them. Wash your hands thoroughly after removing gloves.

When an infectious disease, such as influenza, or one that weakens the immune system, such as AIDS or cancer, is present in the home, take these extra housecleaning precautions:

- Use disinfectant to clean countertops and surfaces in the kitchen and bathroom.

- Clean the bathroom daily. Have other family members use a different bathroom if possible.

- Use separate dishes and utensils for the infected person. In some cases, disposable dishes and utensils should be used.

- Wash dishes and utensils in the dishwasher (Fig. 5-23). Dishes may also be washed in hot soapy water with bleach, rinsed in boiling water, and allowed to air dry.

- Disinfect any surfaces that contact body fluids, such as bedpans, urinals and toilets.

- Frequently remove trash containing used tissues.

- Keep any specimens of urine, stool, or sputum in double bags and away from food or food preparation areas.

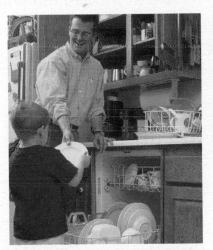

Fig. 5-23. Wash dishes used by an infected person with hot soapy water or in the dishwasher.

When infectious disease is present in the home, take these special precautions when handling laundry:

- Keep laundry separate from that of other family members.

- Wear gloves and hold the laundry away from your clothes and body when you are handling soiled laundry and linens (Fig. 5-24).

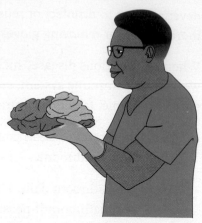

Fig. 5-24. Wear gloves when handling dirty laundry and hold it away from your body.

- Handle dirty laundry as little as possible. Sort it and put it in plastic bags in the infected person's room or bathroom and take it immediately to the laundry area.

- Use liquid bleach when fabrics allow.

- Use Lysol™ or other disinfectants in all loads.

- Use hot water.

Resources

The CDC's website has information on a great number of health topics, including infection control, vaccinations, and individual diseases such as HIV/AIDS and tuberculosis.

Centers for Disease Control and Prevention (CDC)
1600 Clifton Rd
Atlanta, GA 30333

Tel: 800-311-3435
www.cdc.gov

This is a non-profit organization dedicated to the prevention of HIV infection and improving the lives of those with HIV/AIDS.

AIDS.ORG
7985 Santa Monica Blvd, #99
West Hollywood, CA 90046
www.aids.org

The World Health Organization (WHO) is an agency developed by the United Nations to address world health concerns. Their site includes information about specific diseases, including HIV/AIDS.

World Health Organization (WHO)
Avenue Appia 20
1211 Geneva 27
Switzerland
Tel: (+ 41 22) 791 21 11
Fax: (+ 41 22) 791 3111
www.who.int

The Gay Men's Health Crisis is a non-profit organization dedicated to the fight against HIV/AIDS and promoting dignity for gay men and lesbians.

Gay Men's Health Crisis
The Tisch Building
119 West 24th Street
New York, NY 10011
Tel: 212-367-1000
www.gmhc.org

Hepatitis Foundation International offers resources and support to those living with hepatitis and information about hepatitis prevention.

Hepatitis Foundation International
504 Blick Drive
Silver Spring, MD 20904-2901
Tel: 800-891-0707
www.hepfi.org

The American Lung Association has information about tuberculosis and other lung disorders.

The American Lung Association
61 Broadway, 6th Floor
NY, NY 10006
Tel: 800-LUNGUSA
www.lungusa.org

6

Normal and Abnormal Signs of Aging

Because later adulthood covers an age range of as many as 25 to 35 years, people in this age category will have very different capabilities, depending on their health. Some 70-year-old people enjoy active sports, while others are not active. Many 85-year-old people can live alone, while others may live with family members or in nursing homes.

Generalizations or stereotypes about older people are often false, and they create prejudices against the elderly that are as unfair as prejudices against racial, ethnic, or religious groups. On television and in the movies, older people are often shown as helpless, lonely, disabled, slow, forgetful, dependent, or inactive. However, research indicates that most older people are active and engaged in work, volunteer activities, learning programs, and exercise regimens (Fig. 6-1). Aging is a normal process, not a disease. Most older people live independent lives and are able to manage without assistance.

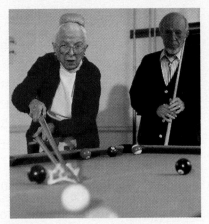

Fig. 6-1. Many older adults remain active and engaged as they age.

For most older adults, the greatest challenge of aging is the need to adjust to change. As personal, physical, social, and work lives change, older adults must become more flexible. The ability to adjust to change, as well as maintaining good physical health, will help older adults continue to live independently and happily.

First Steps

Make yourself aware of the normal signs of aging in the human body. Observe your loved one carefully for changes that could indicate illness.

Remind yourself to encourage your loved one to be as independent as possible. Encourage him to take part in enjoyable activities and to do as many ADLs for himself as possible, even if this takes a long time.

Be alert to your loved one's changing condition and adapt as necessary. Consult the doctor if there are changes that may indicate illness or if you need advice on how to adapt conditions in the home for your aging loved one.

Aging is a continuous process from birth to death. Each person ages in a unique way, influenced by genetics and lifestyle. Although we cannot choose our genetic makeup, we do choose the lifestyle we lead. Early habits of diet, exercise, attitude, social and physical activities, and health maintenance affect our well-being later in life.

An aging parent may need assistance with activities of daily living, such as eating, dressing, and using the bathroom. A person who is chronically ill and needs a lot of help still benefits from living at home. As a caregiver, you are giving a priceless gift by letting your loved one stay in familiar surroundings while getting the help she needs. Being able to distinguish between normal changes of aging and signs of illness will help you provide better care. The following pages explain normal, age-related changes for each body system and related care guidelines.

Integumentary System (Skin)

Changes: Skin is thinner, drier, and more fragile. Much of the fatty layer beneath the skin is lost, causing the person to feel colder. Texture of hair may change. Hair thins and turns gray.

Nails are harder and more brittle. Reduced circulation to the skin can cause dryness, itching, and irritation.

Care:

- Dry skin can become more irritated and itchy if an older person takes tub baths too often. Older adults perspire less and do not need to bathe as frequently. Most elderly people generally need a complete bath only twice a week, with sponge baths every day.

- Moisturizing lotions can help relieve dry skin. Be gentle when assisting with personal care; elderly skin can be fragile and tear easily.

- Hair also becomes drier and needs to be shampooed less often. Gently brush dry hair to stimulate and distribute the natural oils (Fig. 6-2).

- Layer clothing and bed covers for additional warmth.

- Encourage fluids.

Musculoskeletal System (Muscles and Bones)

Changes: Muscles weaken and lose tone. Bones become more brittle, making them easy to break. Joints may stiffen and become painful. Body movement slows. There is a gradual loss of height.

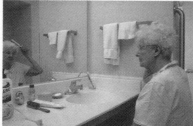

Fig. 6-2. Brushing dry hair helps stimulate and distribute natural oils.

Care:

- To prevent further loss of physical and mental capabilities, encourage your loved one to do as much for himself as he can. The doctor may suggest some range of motion (ROM) exercises that you can assist with. Encourage eating in the kitchen and walking to the bathroom, for example, until these activities are no longer possible. Encourage your loved one to make decisions and dress independently, with assistance if necessary, no matter how long it takes.

- To prevent or slow osteoporosis, the condition that is responsible for fragile bones, encourage walking and other light exercise (Fig. 6-3). Exercise can strengthen bones as well as muscles.

- Falls can cause life-threatening complications, including fractures. Prevent falls by keeping items out of pathways. Always keep furniture in the same place. Keep walkers and canes within easy reach.

Nervous System

Changes: Aging affects the ability to think logically and quickly. How much ability is lost depends on the individual. Aging can also affect

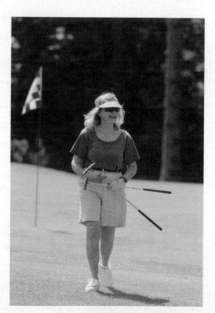

Fig. 6-3. Light exercise can help to prevent or slow osteoporosis.

concentration and memory. Older adults may experience memory loss of recent events. This short-term memory loss may cause anxiety. Long-term memory, or memory for past events, usually remains sharp, and many elderly people enjoy reminiscing, or talking about the past.

Care:

- You may be able to help your loved one with memory retention. Suggest making lists or writing notes about things to remember. Keeping a calendar or clock nearby may help with orientation to date and time.

- If your loved one enjoys reminiscing, show your interest in her past experiences by asking to see photos or hear stories (Fig. 6-4).

- Older people are still able to learn and enjoy new activities, although they sometimes do not learn as quickly as

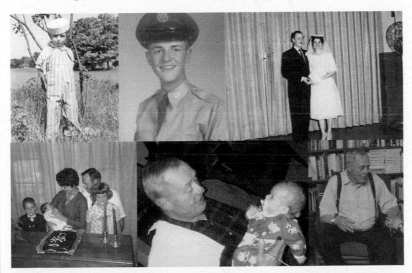

Fig. 6-4. If your loved one enjoys reminiscing, ask to see photos or hear stories. Many people have had rich lives with wonderful experiences.

younger adults. Finding new hobbies or activities can be very beneficial for older adults.

- Encourage reading, thinking, and other mental activities.

- Allow time for decision-making and avoid sudden changes in schedule.

Your loved one may also experience changes in vision, hearing, taste, and smell. The failing vision of many elderly people may make some activities, such as reading, difficult or impossible. Hearing impairment may make it frustrating for older adults to try to communicate. Weakened senses of smell, taste, and touch may present dangers for older adults.

Care:

- Many books and some magazines are available printed in large type. Books on cassette or CD are available at libraries and bookstores.

- Keep eyeglasses clean. Bright colors and good light will also help with poor eyesight (Fig. 6-5). Sometimes eyes do not adapt quickly to glare or to changes from light to dark. If glare is a problem, encourage using sunglasses outdoors. When going into another room, be sure the lights are on before your loved one enters.

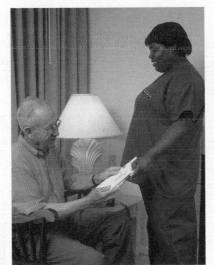

Fig. 6-5. Good lighting will help if your loved one is visually impaired.

- If hearing is a problem, speak in a low-pitched voice; for some people, low-pitched sounds are easier to hear. You may also need to repeat words. Some people need hearing aids and should be encouraged to use them. Keep hearing aids clean. Excess earwax can make hearing difficult; if you suspect excess earwax, tell the doctor or nurse.

- If your loved one has difficulty hearing, face her and speak slowly, simply, and clearly. Do not shout.

- Because we lose taste buds as we age, older people often cannot taste as well as younger people. Decreased sense of smell may contribute to the altered sense of taste. Make sure the food in the house is fresh, because an older person may not be able to smell or taste that food is spoiled. Older people should always have smoke and carbon monoxide detectors in their homes, particularly since they may not smell leaking gas or smoke.

- The sense of touch is also affected by aging. Be careful with hot drinks and hot bath water. Older adults sometimes cannot tell if something is too hot. The elderly person who is confined to bed may not feel uncomfortable, but because of decreased circulation and dry skin, he is at risk for developing pressure sores, sometimes called decubitus ulcers, or bedsores (Fig. 6-6). The sense of pain may also be diminished in the elderly. Always be alert to changes in your loved one's health.

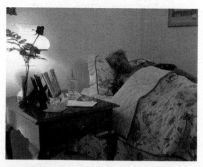

Fig. 6-6. A person confined to bed is at risk for pressure sores.

Disorientation, or confusion about time and place, may occur in new surroundings or as a result of infection or medication. Disorientation is **not** a normal part of aging. Disorientation caused by medication is called drug intoxication. Many elderly people take one or more kinds of medication. Taking the wrong amount or combination of medications can cause disorientation. See chapter 14 for more information on medications.

Care:

- As with all changes in health, always report any observations you make about decreased senses to the doctor. Disorientation may be a sign of illness. Techniques for working with someone who is confused can be found in chapter 9.

Circulatory System

Changes: As we age, our hearts pump less efficiently. Increased activity places greater demands on the heart, which it may not be able to meet. Older people may need more rest to reduce demands on the heart. They may not be able to walk long distances, climb stairs, or exert themselves. Less efficient circulation of blood causes older adults to be more sensitive to the cold.

Care:

- Moderate exercise is necessary and helpful. Walking, stretching, and even lifting light weights can help older people maintain strength and mobility.

- Active or passive range of motion (ROM) exercises are important for those who cannot get out of bed. The doctor or physical therapist will specify the kinds of exercise or activity your loved one should be doing.

- Someone with a heart condition, particularly heart failure, must avoid vigorous activity or exercise, including carrying heavy objects. Some older people may experience dizziness when they stand up too quickly. Encourage rising slowly and standing still for a few moments and holding on to a chair or other piece of furniture for support (Fig. 6-7).

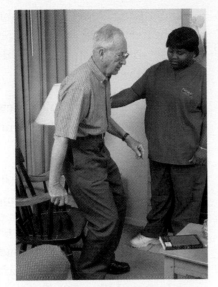

Fig. 6-7. If your loved one gets dizzy when standing up, encourage him to rise slowly and use furniture for support.

- The home may need to be kept at a higher temperature than normally preferred, and older people may need to wear layers of clothing to keep warm. Some elderly adults who are concerned about the cost of heating may lower the thermostat to a dangerous level.

- Poor circulation in the extremities causes the feet to feel cold. Be sure your loved one wears slippers or shoes and socks.

- Do not use hot water bottles or heating pads. Poor circulation causes dry skin that is fragile and can burn easily. In addition, because of the dulled sense of pain, an older person may not realize he is being burned until it is too late.

Respiratory System

Changes: As the body ages, the lungs have fewer alveoli in which oxygen/carbon dioxide exchange can take place. Shortness of breath is a common problem for older adults. Older people may also have a harder time coughing up mucus. The strength and capacity of the lungs and the amount of oxygen in the blood are decreased. The voice is weakened.

Care:

- You may need to provide frequent rest periods when assisting with care.

- Follow instructions for exercise and activity carefully. As noted above in guidelines associated with the circulatory system, moderate exercise is helpful, but overdoing it can be very dangerous for an older adult.

- Encourage and assist with deep breathing exercises.

Urinary System

Changes: The bladder is not able to hold as much urine as it did previously. Older adults may need to urinate more frequently (Fig. 6-8). Many elderly persons awaken several times during the night to urinate. The bladder may not empty completely, causing greater susceptibility to infection.

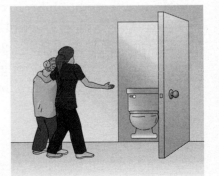

Fig. 6-8. Older adults may need to urinate more frequently.

Care:

- Encourage your loved one to drink plenty of fluids during the day. Offer frequent trips to the bathroom.

- Incontinence is **not** a normal part of aging. Those who are incontinent may need bladder retraining or may wear incontinence pads or briefs. Always report incontinence to the doctor. It may be the symptom of an illness. Cleanliness and good skin care are important for someone who is incontinent. Assist with or teach good perineal care, including wiping from front to back. A urinary catheter may be prescribed to treat incontinence. Special care is needed in this case. Care for someone with a catheter is discussed in chapter 11.

Gastrointestinal System

Changes: Older people who cannot get around easily or who live alone may skip meals or eat foods that are not nutritious. A dulled sense of taste, often made worse by side effects of medications, may result in a poor appetite. Decreased saliva production affects the ability to chew and swallow. Digestion takes longer and is less efficient in older adults. Many older adults have trouble with indigestion, or upset stomach. Body waste moves more slowly through the intestines; constipation, or the inability to have a bowel movement, may occur.

Care:

- Encourage fluids and nutritious, appealing meals. Diet should contain fiber and plenty of fluids to prevent constipation. See chapter 12 for more information on nutrition and meal preparation.

- Older people may have trouble chewing because of loose dentures, dental problems, or gum disease, and may require soft foods. Make sure dentures fit properly and are cleaned regularly.

- People who have trouble chewing and swallowing are at risk of choking. Provide plenty of fluids with meals. Cut food into bite-sized pieces.

- Some older adults need to eat several small meals a day or have the large meal in the middle of the day.

Dehydration is a condition that results from inadequate fluid in the body. It is not a normal sign of aging; however, many older people do not feel thirsty and may not be aware that they are dehydrated (Fig. 6-9). Dehydration can cause constipation, weight loss, dry skin, infection, dizziness and weakness, and other illnesses that require medical attention.

Care:

- Encourage your loved one to drink regularly. Offer fresh water or other fluids often.

- Ice chips, frozen flavored ice sticks, and gelatin are also forms of liquids. Offer them often. Do not offer ice chips or sticks if your loved one has a swallowing problem.

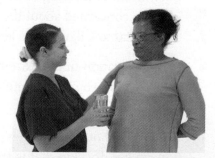

Fig. 6-9. Some older people do not feel thirsty and may not be aware that they are dehydrated.

- Offer sips of liquid between bites of food at meals and snacks.

- Make sure a pitcher and cup are nearby and are light enough for your loved one to lift.

- Offer assistance if your loved one cannot drink without help.

- You may be asked to measure fluid intake and output. Measure and document carefully to ensure that fluid balance is healthy. You will learn how to monitor fluid balance in chapter 12.

Endocrine System

Changes: Levels of reproductive hormones are lower. Pancreas function lessens, which may lead to diabetes for some people.

Care:

- Older people may need to take insulin or eat certain foods to regulate blood sugar. The doctor or nurse will provide instruction. More information on diabetes is in chapter 7.

Reproductive System

Changes: Genital areas may become dry and uncomfortable. In males, the prostate gland increases in size. In females, fatty tissue in the breasts may diminish, and mucous secretions in the vagina decrease. Though the reproductive organs change, sexual needs and desires do not necessarily change.

Care:

- Avoiding too many hot baths can help prevent discomfort in the genital area.

- Despite changes in the reproductive organs, older adults remain sexual beings (Fig. 6-10). Allow as much privacy as possible while still providing good care. It is best not to make any assumptions or generalizations about the sexual feelings of older adults.

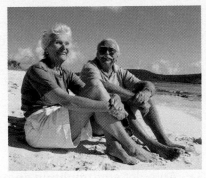

Fig. 6-10. Human beings continue to have sexual needs throughout their lives.

- Do be aware of behavior that seems inappropriate. Inappropriate behavior is not a normal sign of aging, and could be a sign of illness.

Immune and Lymphatic Systems

Changes: As we age, our immune system gradually weakens. It may take longer to recover from an illness. Bone marrow activity (which produces white blood cells that fight infections) decreases as we age. Changes in the respiratory system's protective surface may result in increased respiratory infections. The number and size of lymph nodes is reduced. This results in the body being less able to contract a fever to fight infection.

Many elderly people develop anemia, especially iron-deficiency anemia, due to poor nutrition and less efficient use of nutrients by the body. While anemia is common, it is **not** a normal sign of aging. Report to the doctor any signs and symptoms of anemia, including weakness, fainting, light-headedness, and headache.

Care:

- Vaccines against common infections, such as influenza (flu), are very important for older adults. Ask your doctor about which vaccines might be beneficial for your loved one.

- Encourage proper nutrition and fluid intake to help older adults stay healthy.

- An older adult fighting an infection may not experience a fever. Even a slight temperature increase may indicate that the person is fighting an infection. Taking accurate vital signs is very important, especially with older adults. You will learn how to take vital signs in chapter 11.

Psychological Changes

Some forgetfulness is a normal part of aging, but constant memory lapses or forgetting basic information, such as the names of family members, are not normal changes of aging.

Care:

Any of the following signs should be reported to the doctor, as they may indicate illness:

- disorientation, or change in ability to remember who he is, what month or season of the year it is, or other basic facts

- difficulty concentrating

- depression

- dementia, or a loss of mental abilities that interferes with daily life

- confusion

- suicidal thoughts

- insomnia or inability to sleep

Depression is very common among the elderly, but it is not a normal sign of aging. Elderly persons may not admit feelings of depression to themselves or others. According to the National Center for Health Statistics, the elderly are at higher risk for suicide than all other age groups. Be alert for any signs of depression. In many cases, depression can be successfully treated.

Care:

- Observing and reporting signs and symptoms is the best way to help someone who may be suffering from depression. Signs and symptoms of depression include anorexia, or loss of appetite; insomnia, or difficulty sleeping; acting moody or withdrawn; and other changes in appearance, speech, movement, and behavior. Sleep disorders and emotional changes, such as hopelessness; anxiety; apathy, or lack of interest; agitation; restlessness; and demanding or violent behavior are particularly important to report.

Lifestyle Changes

Aging brings many social, physical, and mental changes. Friends, colleagues, and relatives die; physical strength and stamina diminish; and fears of illness, injury, and death may increase. Retirement causes changes in what and how much people do each day. Living arrangements may also change. These changes require adjustment, which can become more difficult as people age.

Care:

- You can help your loved one adjust to change by listening to her and caring about her feelings (Fig. 6-11).

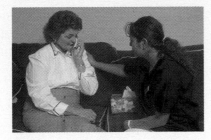

Fig. 6-11. You can help your loved one adjust to change by listening to her.

- Ensuring that she is safe is another way you help her adapt to her changing lifestyle. Chapter 4 describes ways to make the home safer for an elderly or frail person.

The psychological and social needs of older adults are the same as those of younger people. The needs for love and affection, acceptance by others, and interaction with other people do not go away with age. Staying active, maintaining self-esteem, and living independently can promote good physical and mental health for older adults. Encourage your loved one to pursue activities he enjoys and can succeed in (Fig. 6-12).

Many older people enjoy reading, playing checkers, playing cards, doing crafts, or listening to music. Working with others on charity or community service projects can allow older people to

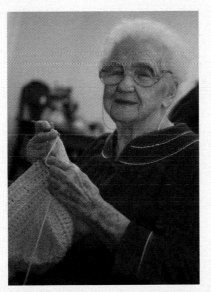

Fig. 6-12. Encourage your loved one to pursue enjoyable activities.

share their knowledge and experience. Senior centers or community centers offer classes, hobby groups, and field trips that some older adults may enjoy. Many older people are involved in activities through a church or synagogue.

Develop a routine for the day. Structuring the day around meals, activities, rest, and self-care can help fight depression and give older adults a sense of purpose. Older people who don't have a routine may simply stay in bed or become bored and lonely.

Encourage self-care. Your loved one should do as much for herself as she possibly can. You won't be helping her by giving her a bath if that is something she could do for herself. Assist with or perform only activities she cannot do alone. The more she can care for herself, the better she will feel about herself.

Help your loved one to be well groomed (Fig. 6-13). Appearance affects the way we feel about ourselves. Help with styling hair, dressing neatly, using cosmetics, or shaving.

Ask for your loved one's opinions and let him make his own decisions as often as possible. The more independent and capable he feels, the more independent and capable he will be. Never treat an older person like a

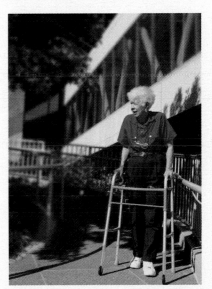

Fig. 6-13. A well-groomed appearance helps a person feel good about herself.

child or talk about him as if he were not in the room.

Respect your loved one's needs for privacy and for social interaction. Let her be alone to read, study, pray, or work if she seems to want this. Knock before you enter the room, even if the door is open (Fig. 6-14). Encourage visitors if they lift your loved one's spirits.

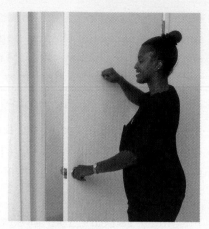

Fig. 6-14. Always knock before entering your loved one's room.

Resources

This site offers mental health information and information about clinical trials and research being conducted in the field of mental health.

National Institute of Mental Health (NIMH)
Office of Communications
6001 Executive Boulevard, Room 8184, MSC 9663
Bethesda, MD 20892-9663
Tel: 301-443-4513
Toll-free: 866-615-6464
TTY: 301-443-8431
Fax: 301-443-4279
www.nimh.nih.gov

The CDC's healthy aging site promotes health and quality of life for aging persons as well as disease prevention. This page also has a link to an alphabetized list of health topics and relevant information.

Centers for Disease Control and Prevention (CDC)
Healthy Aging for Older Adults
E-mail comments or questions to ccdinfo@cdc.gov
www.cdc.gov/aging

This comprehensive site from the U.S. National Library of Medicine and the National Institutes of Health has information on over 700 health topics. There is also a link to information about prescription and over-the-counter medications, a medical encyclopedia, and a dictionary of medical terms.

MedLine Plus
U.S. National Library of Medicine
8600 Rockville Pike
Bethesda, MD 20894
Tel: 888-346-3656
www.medlineplus.gov

Meeting Special Needs and Conditions

There are a number of reasons you may find yourself caring for someone in your home. Whether your loved one has been injured in an accident, is recovering from surgery, or is close to death, much of the information in this book will be helpful to you. In this chapter, we will discuss specific situations and offer information and suggestions particular to some of the common conditions found in home care.

First Steps

Find organizations that can provide information and support for the special needs of you and your loved one. Look at the resources listed in this book, online, or in your local telephone book.

Arrange for a healthcare professional to teach you any tests and procedures that you will need to do regularly, such as testing the blood glucose level of a diabetic person or performing ostomy care. See later in the chapter for information on ostomy care.

Ask a healthcare professional to come to your home and help you adapt it to your needs, such as making a safe area for a person with dementia to wander in. This will need to be done periodically as your loved one's condition and needs change.

Arthritis

Arthritis is a general term for inflammation of the joints that causes stiffness, pain, and decreased mobility. Arthritis may occur due to aging, injury, or an autoimmune illness in which the immune system attacks normal tissue in the body. There are several types of arthritis.

Osteoarthritis is a common type of arthritis that affects many elderly people. Osteoarthritis may occur with aging or as the result of joint injury. It commonly affects the hips and knees, which are weight-bearing joints. Joints of the fingers, thumbs, and spine may also be affected. Pain and stiffness seem to increase in cold or damp weather.

Rheumatoid arthritis affects people of all ages. Physicians believe that an infection activates the immune system's inflammatory response, causing attacks on normal connective tissue in the joints and throughout the body. The joints become inflamed, red, swollen, and very painful; movement is eventually restricted (Fig. 7-1). Fever, fatigue, and weight loss are also symptoms. Rheumatoid arthritis usually affects the small joints first, then progresses to larger ones. The heart, lungs, eyes, kidneys, and skin may also be affected.

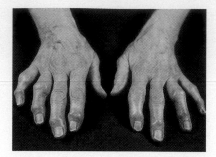

Fig. 7-1. Rheumatoid arthritis. (Photo courtesy of Frederick Miller, MD)

Arthritis is generally treated with some or all of the following:

- anti-inflammatory medications such as aspirin or ibuprofen

- local applications of heat to reduce swelling and pain

- range of motion exercises

- a regular exercise and/or activity regimen

- diet to reduce weight or maintain strength

GUIDELINES
Arthritis

Watch for stomach irritation or heartburn caused by aspirin or ibuprofen. Some people cannot tolerate these medications. Report signs of stomach irritation immediately.

Encourage activity. Gentle activity can help reduce the effects of arthritis. Use canes or other walking aids as needed.

Adapt activities of daily living to allow independence. Many devices are available to allow people to bathe, dress, and feed themselves even when arthritis has impaired their abilities (Fig. 7-2). Choose clothing that is easy to put on and fasten. Install handrails and safety bars in the bathroom. Special utensils are available to make eating easier.

Help maintain morale. Although arthritis is common, it is a chronic, painful, degenerative disease which can have devastating effects. By encouraging self-care, maintaining a positive attitude, and listening to her feelings, you can help your loved one manage the disease and remain independent for as long as possible.

Cancer

Cancer is a general term used to describe many types of malignant tumors. A tumor is a cluster of abnormally growing cells. Benign tumors grow slowly in local areas and are considered noncancerous. Malignant tumors grow rapidly and invade surrounding tissues.

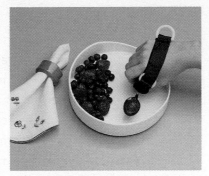

Fig. 7-2. Special equipment can help a person with arthritis remain independent. (Photo courtesy of North Coast Medical, Inc., 800-821-9319 www.ncmedical.com)

Cancer often appears first in the breast, colon, rectum, uterus, prostate, lungs, or skin. It can not only invade local tissue, but it can spread, or metastasize, to other parts of the body. When a cancer has metastasized, it has spread from the site where it first appeared to affect one or more other body systems. This process is called metastasis. In general, treatment is more difficult and cancer is more deadly after metastasis has occurred.

Although many advances in cancer research have been made in the past twenty years, there is no known cure for cancer. Cancer appears to overwhelm the body's immune system when tumors grow too large or develop in areas of the body that cannot be reached by the infection-fighting cells of the immune system. However, some treatments (discussed below) are effective.

When diagnosed early, cancer can often be treated and controlled. The American Cancer Society has identified seven warning signs of cancer.

The American Cancer Society's Seven Warning Signs of Cancer:

1. Change in bowel or bladder habits

2. A sore that does not heal

3. Unusual bleeding or discharge from a body opening

4. Thickening or lump in the breast or elsewhere

5. Indigestion or difficulty swallowing

6. Obvious change in a wart or mole

7. Nagging cough or persistent hoarseness

People with cancer can often live longer and can sometimes recover if they are treated with the following methods. These treatments are most effective when tumors are discovered early. Often these treatments are used in combination.

1. Surgery is the first line of defense for most forms of cancer and is the key treatment for malignant tumors of the skin, breast, bladder, colon, rectum, stomach, and muscle. Surgeons attempt to remove as much of the tumor as possible to prevent cancer from spreading.

2. Chemotherapy refers to medications given to fight cancer. Drugs have been developed to destroy cancer cells and limit the rate of cell growth. However, many of these drugs are toxic to the body and destroy healthy cells as well as cancer cells. Chemotherapy can have severe side effects, including nausea, vomiting, diarrhea, hair loss, and decreased resistance to infection.

3. Radiation kills normal as well as abnormal cells. Radiation therapy directs radiation to a limited area to kill only cancer cells, but other cells in its path are also destroyed (Fig. 7-3). By controlling cell growth, radiation can reduce pain. Radiation can cause the same side effects as chemotherapy. The skin of the area exposed to radiation may become sore, irritated, and sometimes burned.

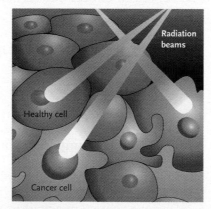

Fig. 7-3. Radiation is targeted at cancer cells, but it also destroys some healthy cells in its path.

GUIDELINES
Cancer

Nutrition. Good nutrition is extremely important for the person with cancer. Follow the doctor's instructions carefully. In general, a person with cancer needs many calories and should be served four to six meals a day. Serve favorite foods that are high in nutrition. Some doctors recommend serving fluids between meals instead of with meals so more food can be eaten. Liquid nutrition supplements may also be used in addition to, but not in place of, meals. If nausea or swallowing is a problem, try to find foods such as soups, gelatin, or starches that may be appealing. Use plastic utensils to make food taste better for someone who is receiving chemotherapy; metal utensils cause a bitter taste.

Pain control. Cancer can cause terrible pain, especially in the late stages. Watch for signs of pain. Observe the use of pain medication. Provide comfort if possible by repositioning and offering distractions such as conversation, music, or reading materials (Fig. 7-4).

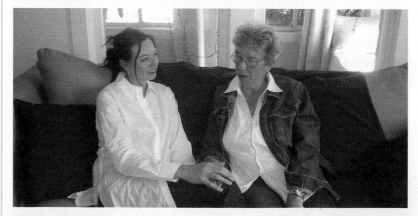

Fig. 7-4. Distractions such as conversation can help a person with cancer deal with pain.

Skin care. Use lotion regularly on dry or delicate skin. Do not apply lotion to areas receiving radiation therapy. Offer back rubs to give comfort and increase circulation. For those who spend many hours in bed, egg crate mattress covers or sheepskins may be more comfortable. Moving to a chair for some period of time may improve comfort as well. Someone who is very weak or immobile needs to be repositioned every two hours.

Oral care. Help your loved one brush and floss his teeth regularly. Medications, nausea, vomiting, or mouth infections such as thrush may cause a bad taste in the mouth. Persons receiving chemotherapy are at risk for oral discomfort. Using a soft-bristled toothbrush or a sponge swab, rinsing with baking soda and water, or using a prescribed rinse can help ease discomfort. Do not use a commercial mouthwash, as alcohol can further irritate the mouth.

Odor control. People suffering from cancer, especially in the late stages, may have an unpleasant odor at times. You can use a room deodorizer to mask any odor you notice. However, you should check with your loved one before using a deodorizer, as a new smell may trigger or worsen nausea.

Self-image. People with cancer may suffer from a low self-image because they are weak and their appearance has changed (for example, hair loss is a common side effect of chemotherapy). Help your loved one feel more attractive by helping her to bathe and dress and offering hats or scarves to cover her head.

Psychosocial needs. If visitors help cheer your loved one, encourage them. If some times of day are better than others, suggest this to friends or family. Support groups exist for people with cancer and their families. Check at the hospital or doctor's office for referrals in your area. It may help a person with cancer to think of something besides cancer and treatment for a while; pursue other topics. As always, report any signs of depression to the doctor.

Caregiver stress. Caring for a person with cancer at home can be very difficult for you. Be alert to your own needs and to stresses created by the illness. Try to give yourself the breaks you need. Know the resources available in your area.

Numerous services and support groups are available for people with cancer and their families or caregivers. Hospitals, hospice programs, churches, and synagogues offer many resources, including meal services, transportation to doctors' offices or hospitals, counseling, and support groups. Check the local yellow pages under "cancer" or call the local or state chapter of the American Cancer Society and your local Area Agency on Aging.

Ostomies

An ostomy is surgical removal of a portion of the intestines. The end of the intestine is brought out of the body through an artificial opening in the abdomen, called a stoma. Feces is eliminated through the stoma rather than through the anus. People with cancer or bowel disease or accident victims may require ostomies. The terms "colostomy" and "ileostomy" indicate which section of the intestine was removed and the type of stool that will be eliminated. In a colostomy, stool will generally be semi-solid. With an ileostomy, stool may be liquid and irritating to the skin.

If your loved one has had an ostomy, she will wear a disposable bag that fits over the stoma to collect the feces. The bag is attached to her skin by adhesive; it may also be secured by a belt. These devices are called the ostomy appliance (Fig. 7-5).

Adapting to wearing an ostomy appliance can be difficult or upsetting for some people. They feel they have lost control of a basic function, and they are embarrassed or angry. It is important to be sensitive and to provide privacy along with whatever help is needed for care of an ostomy. Remember to use good infection control and hygiene procedures with ostomy care; wear gloves, wash your hands, and disinfect surfaces that may become contaminated.

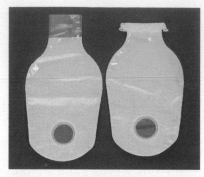

Fig. 7-5. Open and closed ostomy appliances.

Caring for an ostomy

Equipment: bedpan, disposable bed protector, bath blanket, clean ostomy bag and belt/appliance, toilet paper, basin of warm water, soap or cleanser, washcloth, skin cream as ordered, two towels, plastic trash bag or old newspaper, disposable gloves

1   Wash your hands.

2   Discuss what you will do.

3   Provide privacy.

4   Place the protective sheet under your loved one. Cover him with a bath blanket. Have him hold the bath blanket while you pull down the top sheet and blankets. Expose ostomy site. Offer him a towel to keep clothing dry.

5   Put on gloves.

6   Remove the ostomy bag carefully. If it will be washed and reused, place it in the bedpan. If it will be discarded, wrap it in newspaper or the plastic trash bag. Note the color, odor, consistency, and amount of stool in the bag.

7   Wipe the area around the stoma with toilet paper. Discard paper in bedpan.

8   Using a washcloth and warm soapy water, wash the area around the stoma (Fig. 7-6). Pat dry with another towel. Apply cream as ordered.

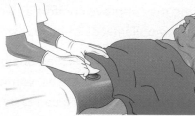

Fig. 7-6.

9   Place the clean ostomy appliance on your loved one, following instructions. Make sure the bottom of the bag is clamped.

10   Remove the plastic protector sheet and discard.

11   Remove gloves. Make your loved one comfortable. Put on fresh gloves and change linens if necessary. Cover him and remove bath blanket and towel.

12   Put on a new pair of gloves. Take bedpan and other supplies to bathroom. Empty bag into toilet and flush, along with used toilet paper. Wash out bag and use a deodorant in the bag as directed.

13   Wash out the bedpan and store. Clean basin and store.

14   Remove gloves.

15   Wash your hands.

16   Note any observations.
Note: Call the doctor if stoma appears very red or blue, or if swelling or bleeding is present.

Diabetes

In diabetes mellitus, commonly called diabetes, the pancreas does not produce enough insulin. Insulin is the substance the body needs to convert glucose, or natural sugar, into energy. If insulin is not present to process glucose, it accumulates in the blood, causing problems with circulation and possibly damaging vital organs.

Diabetes commonly occurs in people with a family history of the illness, in the elderly, and in people who are obese. Two types of diabetes have been identified:

Type 1 diabetes is usually diagnosed in children and young adults; it was formerly known as juvenile diabetes. It most often appears before age 20. In type 1 diabetes, the body does not produce insulin. The condition will continue throughout a person's life. A person can develop type 1 diabetes up to age 40. Type 1 diabetes is treated with insulin and diet.

Type 2 diabetes is the most common form of diabetes. In type 2 diabetes, either the body does not produce enough insulin or the body fails to properly use insulin. This is known as "insulin resistance." It can usually be controlled with diet and/or oral medications. It is also called adult-onset diabetes. Type 2 diabetes usually develops slowly. It is the milder form of diabetes. It typically develops after age 35; the risk of getting it increases with age. However, the number of children with type 2 diabetes is growing rapidly. Type 2 diabetes often occurs in obese people or those with a family history of the disease.

People with diabetes mellitus may have the following signs and symptoms:

- increased thirst

- increased hunger

- weight loss

- elevated levels of blood sugar

- presence of sugar in the urine

- increased frequency of urination

Diabetes can lead to the following complications:

- Changes in the circulatory system can cause heart attack and stroke, reduced circulation to the extremities, poor wound healing, and kidney and nerve damage.

- Damage to the eyes can cause impaired vision and blindness.

- Poor circulation and impaired wound healing may result in leg and foot ulcers, infected wounds, and gangrene. Gangrene can lead to amputation. Good foot care is vital for people with diabetes (Fig. 7-7).

In some cases, diet modification and an exercise regimen are enough to bring a diabetic person's blood sugar into normal range. However, if blood sugar remains outside the acceptable range, in-

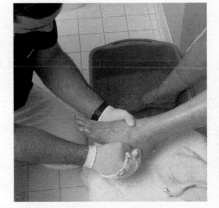

Fig. 7-7. Good foot care, including close observation of the feet, is essential for diabetics.

sulin may be needed to restore and maintain a healthy level. This does not mean that your loved one is not following the meal plan or exercising; it simply indicates that the body is still not producing a healthy amount of insulin. If necessary, the doctor will prescribe insulin injections to bring insulin in the body to a healthy level. You and your loved one may be asked to see a nurse educator who will teach you how, where, and when to administer the insulin injections. Even if your loved one already knows how to administer his insulin, it is a good idea for you to learn as well.

Insulin can be stored at room temperature or in the refrigerator. Cold insulin tends to be painful when injected; if it is kept in the refrigerator, let it sit at room temperature for 15 minutes before injection. Insulin should be stored away from extreme heat or cold. The expiration date on the label is applicable if the bottle has never been opened; once opened, the bottle is only good for 28 days. Write the date that the bottle was opened on the label and check it frequently to ensure that you do not use it after 28 days.

Insulin shock and diabetic coma are complications of diabetes that can be life-threatening. Insulin shock, or hypoglycemia, can result from either too much insulin or too little food. It frequently occurs when a dose of insulin is administered and the person skips a meal or does not eat all the food required. Even when a regular amount of food is eaten, excessive physical activity may rapidly metabolize the food so that the amount of insulin in the body is excessive. Vomiting and diarrhea may also lead to insulin shock in people with diabetes.

The first signs of insulin shock include feeling weak or "different," nervousness, dizziness, and perspiration (see list below for further signs). These are signals that the person needs food in a form that can be rapidly absorbed. A lump of sugar, a hard candy, or a glass of orange juice should be consumed right away. Someone who is diabetic should always have a quick source of sugar handy.

The following are signs and symptoms of insulin shock:

- hunger
- weakness
- rapid pulse
- headache
- low blood pressure
- perspiration
- cold, clammy skin
- confusion
- trembling
- nervousness
- blurred vision
- numbness of the lips and tongue
- unconsciousness

Diabetic coma, also known as acidosis or hyperglycemia, is caused by having too little insulin. It can result from undiagnosed diabetes, going without insulin or not taking enough, eating too much food, not getting enough exercise, and physical or emotional stress.

The signs of diabetic coma include increased thirst or urination, abdominal pain, deep or labored breathing, and breath that smells sweet or fruity (see complete list of symptoms below). Remember that insulin and exercise lower blood sugar and consumption of food raises blood sugar. Call the doctor immediately if you suspect diabetic coma or insulin shock. Discuss with your doctor when to call emergency services.

Other signs and symptoms of diabetic coma include the following:

- hunger
- weakness
- rapid, weak pulse
- headache
- low blood pressure
- dry skin
- flushed cheeks
- drowsiness
- slow, deep, and labored breathing
- nausea and vomiting
- abdominal pain
- sweet, fruity breath odor
- air hunger, or gasping for air and being unable to catch a breath
- unconsciousness

GUIDELINES
Diabetes

Diabetes must be carefully controlled to prevent complications and severe illness. Keep the following guidelines in mind:

Follow diet instructions exactly. The intake of carbohydrates, including breads, potatoes, grains, pasta, and sugars, must be regulated. Meals must be eaten at the same time each day, and your loved one must eat everything that is served. If he refuses to eat what is directed or if you suspect that he is not following the diet, report this and discuss it with the doctor. More information on diet for a person with diabetes is provided later in this chapter.

Be sure your loved one follows an exercise program (Fig. 7-8). Because exercise affects the body's rate of metabolism and the amount of insulin produced by the pancreas, a regular exercise program is important. This may include 30 to 60 minutes of activity on most days of the week. Exercise also helps improve circulation. Exercises may include walking or other active exercise or passive range of motion exercises. Encourage him to perform the exercises provided, and help as necessary. Try to make it fun. A walk can be a chore or it can be the highlight of the day.

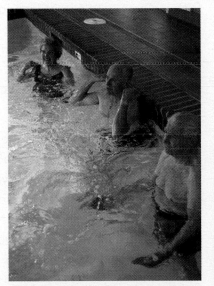

Fig. 7-8. Following an exercise program is very important for diabetics.

Meeting Special Needs and Conditions

7

Observe the management of insulin doses. Doses are calculated exactly and should be administered at the same time each day, or exactly according to instructions.

Perform urine and blood tests as directed. Sometimes the doctor will specify that blood or urine be tested daily to determine sugar or insulin levels (Fig. 7-9).

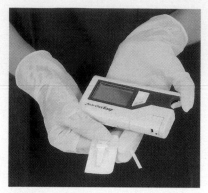

Fig. 7-9. This equipment measures blood glucose levels.

Perform foot care only as directed. Because circulation may be decreased in people with diabetes, they are susceptible to ulcers and sores that may not heal. Even a small sore on the leg or foot can grow into a large wound that could result in amputation. Careful foot care, including inspection, monitoring, and prevention of irritation, is very important for someone with diabetes. The goals of diabetic foot care are to check for signs of irritation or sores, to stimulate blood circulation, and to prevent infection.

In addition to daily foot care, the person with diabetes should be encouraged to wear comfortable, well-fitting shoes that do not irritate or hurt the feet. To avoid cuts or injuries to the feet, a diabetic should never go barefoot. Cotton socks are best because they absorb perspiration. Never attempt to cut the toenails of a person with diabetes yourself. Only a nurse or physician should cut a diabetic's toenails.

People with diabetes must be very careful about what they eat. In order to keep their blood glucose levels near normal, they must eat the right amount of the right type of food at the right time of day. To make it easier to determine what they should be eating, people with diabetes are usually taught to follow meal plans and use exchange lists.

A dietitian should work closely with you or your loved one to make up a meal plan that includes all the right types and amounts of food for each day. Then you can use exchange lists, or lists of similar foods that can substitute for one another, to make up a menu for each day. For example, the meal plan might call for one starch and one fruit to be eaten as a snack. Looking at the exchange list, your loved one can choose which starch and fruit he wants to eat. The list includes many choices, from bagels to biscuits to pretzels. The equivalent serving size for each food is also given, so he will get the right amount of carbohydrates, protein, and fat to meet the meal plan requirements. Using meal plans and exchange lists, a person with diabetes can control his diet while still making his own food choices (Fig. 7-10).

Sample Meal Plan and Exchange List

The following is a sample meal plan and a partial exchange list a person with diabetes might use. Keep in mind that this is only an example. A person's diet may also be under other restrictions. The diet will vary according to the person's daily caloric needs. Actual exchange lists contain many more choices than the sample below.

Sample Meal Plan

- Breakfast (to be eaten between 7:30 and 8:30 a.m.): two starches, one milk, one fruit, one fat

- Snack (to be eaten between 10 and 11 a.m.): one milk

- Lunch (12:30 to 1:30 p.m.): one meat, one milk, two starches, one vegetable, one fruit

- Snack (3:00 to 4:00 p.m.): one vegetable, one milk

- Dinner (5:30 to 6:30 p.m.): three meats, one starch, two vegetables, one milk, two fats

- Snack (7:30 to 8:30 p.m.): one milk, one starch

Following the meal plan for what types of food and how many servings to eat, the person chooses specific foods and determines serving sizes using the exchange lists.

Exchange List Sample Items

- Starch list: 1 slice of bread, 1/2 bagel, 1/2 cup cereal, 1/2 cup pasta, 1/2 cup rice, 1 baked potato, 3 cups popcorn, 15-20 fat-free potato chips

- Milk list: 1 cup milk (skim, 1%, 2%, or whole, depending on other dietary guidelines), 3/4 cup yogurt

- Fruit list: 1/2 cup unsweetened applesauce, 1 small banana, 1/2 cup orange juice, 2 tablespoons raisins, 1 small orange, 1/2 cup canned pears

- Vegetable list: 1/2 cup cooked vegetables or vegetable juice, 1 cup raw vegetables (not included are corn, potatoes, and peas, which are on the starch exchange list instead)

- Meat list: 1 oz. meat, fish, poultry, or cheese, 1 egg, or 1/2 cup dried beans

- Fat list: 1 tsp margarine or butter, 2 tsps peanut butter, 2 tbsps sour cream, 1 tsp mayonnaise, 10 peanuts

Fig. 7-10. A sample meal plan and exchange list.

Cerebral Vascular Accident (CVA)

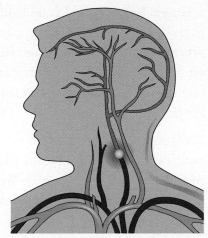

Fig. 7-11. A stroke is caused when the blood supply to the brain is cut off suddenly by a clot or ruptured blood vessel.

The medical term for a stroke is a cerebral vascular accident, or CVA. CVA occurs when blood supply to the brain is cut off suddenly by a clot or a ruptured blood vessel (Fig. 7-11). The section of the brain that was fed by the damaged blood vessel no longer receives oxygen, and cells die. Leaking blood, clots, and swelling cause pressure on surrounding areas of healthy tissue in the brain, creating further damage.

A transient ischemic attack, or TIA, is a warning sign of a CVA. It is the result of a temporary lack of oxygen in the brain. Symptoms may last up to 24 hours. They include tingling, weakness, or some loss of movement in an extremity. These symptoms should not be ignored; report any of them to your doctor immediately.

A stroke may be preceded by symptoms that signal the oncoming hemorrhage or blockage. These symptoms may include dizziness, ringing in the ears, headache, nausea, vomiting, slurring of words, and loss of memory. These symptoms should also be reported immediately.

Signs that a stroke is occurring include any of the following: loss of consciousness, redness in the face, noisy breathing, seizures, loss of bowel and bladder control, hemiplegia, hemiparesis, aphasia, use of inappropriate words, elevated blood pressure, and slow pulse rate. Hemiplegia refers to paralysis on one side of the body. Hemiparesis refers to weakness on one side of the body. Aphasia is the inability to speak or to speak clearly.

Because the two sides of the brain control different functions, the location of the symptoms will indicate the side of the brain in which the stroke occurred. Weaknesses on the right side of the body indicate that the left side of the brain was affected; weaknesses on the left side of the body indicate that the right side of the brain was affected.

Strokes can be mild or severe. After a stroke, a person may experience any of the following:

- weakness or paralysis on one side of the body

- difficulty speaking or inability to speak

- inability to express needs to others through speech or writing

- trouble understanding spoken or written words

- loss of sensations such as temperature or touch

- loss of bowel or bladder control

- confusion

- laughing or crying without any reason or when it is inappropriate

- poor judgment

- memory loss

- loss of cognitive abilities

- tendency to ignore a weak or paralyzed side of the body

- difficulty swallowing

In the case of a mild stroke the person may experience few, if any, of these effects. Physical therapy may help stroke victims regain physical abilities. Speech therapy and occupational therapy can also be useful in helping a person who has had a stroke learn to communicate and perform activities of daily living again.

GUIDELINES
CVA

A person who has had a stroke will need care that is specific to her disabilities. A person with hemiplegia will need different care than someone with speech loss. The following are general guidelines:

A person with paralysis, weakness, or loss of movement will usually receive physical therapy or occupational therapy. You may be asked to participate by helping her perform exercises or try to use her limbs. Range of motion exercises will help strengthen muscles and keep joints mobile. She may also be instructed to perform leg exercises to improve circulation. Safety is always important when exercising after CVA.

When providing personal care for someone with one-sided paralysis or weakness, you will need to adapt the procedures you use. When helping with transfers or walking, stand on the weaker side. Always use a gait belt for safety.

It is not helpful to refer to the weaker side as the "bad side," or to talk about the "bad" leg or arm. There are more neutral terms, such as "weaker" or "involved," to refer to the side with paralysis or paresis, or weakness. Or you can focus on the uninvolved side—the side without weakness or paralysis.

People with speech loss or communication problems may receive speech therapy. You may be asked to help with exercises. These may include helping recognize written or spoken words. Speech therapists will also evaluate swallowing ability to determine if swallowing therapy or thickened liquids are needed.

Use verbal and nonverbal communication to express your positive attitude. Express your confidence in your loved one's abilities through your smiles, touches, and gestures. Gestures and pointing can also help you convey practical information or allow him to speak to you. More ideas for communication after CVA are included later in this chapter.

Experiencing confusion or memory loss is upsetting. Sometimes a stroke will result in changes in thinking and emotions. People often cry for no reason after a stroke. In some cases, multiple strokes can cause a form of dementia similar to the changes that occur in people with Alzheimer's disease. Caring for a person who is confused, upset, or forgetful requires a lot of patience. Again, your positive attitude will be important. Establishing a routine of care will also help make him feel more secure. More information on working with a person with dementia can be found later in this chapter.

Monitoring safety in the home after CVA is essential. Those who are unsteady, weak, or confused are at risk of falling. Older people are often seriously injured by falls because their bones are more fragile. A person with loss of sensation is at risk of burning herself in the bath or shower or at the stove. Some safety tips include:

- Remove any hazards from the home, including unnecessary clutter or throw rugs.

- Unplug appliances, like toasters and coffee makers, when not in use.

- Check the refrigerator and cabinets for spoiled food. A stroke may impair the senses of smell and taste.

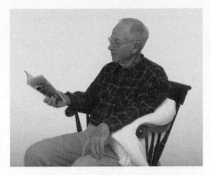

Fig. 7-12. If a person is sitting, place the elbow on an armrest to support a weaker shoulder. This helps keeps the body in proper alignment.

- Follow the instructions for safe transfers using good body mechanics (see chapters 4 and 10).

- Observe body alignment. Sometimes an arm or leg can be caught out of alignment (Fig 7-12).

- Pay special attention to skin care. Watch for changes in the skin if your loved one is unable to move.

Encourage independence and self-esteem. Whatever the effects of the stroke, a person should be encouraged to learn to care for himself again as much as possible. Let him do things for himself whenever possible, even if you could do a better or faster job. Appreciate and acknowledge his efforts to do things independently even when they are unsuccessful. Praise even the smallest successes to build confidence.

After CVA, there is likely to be some degree of weakness on one side of the body. The basic procedures for assisting with transfers (chapter 10) can still be used. However, some additional guidelines must be remembered for everyone's safety.

- Support the involved side.

- Lead with the uninvolved (stronger) side (Fig. 7-13).

- Follow the principles of good body mechanics discussed in chapter 4.

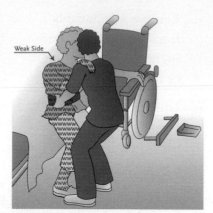
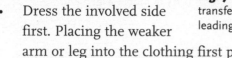

Weak Side

Fig. 7-13. When helping a person transfer, support the weak side while leading with the stronger side.

When assisting your loved one in getting dressed, remember the following:

- Dress the involved side first. Placing the weaker arm or leg into the clothing first prevents unnecessary bending and stretching of the limb.

- Undress the uninvolved side first. Leading with the stronger side and then removing the weaker arm or leg from clothing last prevents the limb from being stretched and twisted to remove the clothing.

- Use adaptive equipment to allow independent dressing.

- Encourage self-care.

When assisting with your loved one with eating, remember the following:

- Be sure to place food within her field of vision (Fig. 7-14).

- Use assistive devices such as silverware with built-up handle grips, plate guards, and drinking cups.

- Watch for signs of choking.

- Serve soft foods if swallowing is difficult.

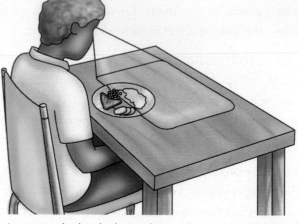

Fig. 7-14. A person who has had a stroke may have a limited field of vision. Make sure your loved one can see what you place in front of him or her.

- Place food in the unaffected side of the mouth. Make sure all food is swallowed before offering more bites.

GUIDELINES

Communicating after CVA

Depending on the severity of the stroke and the degree of speech loss or confusion, the following tips may be helpful:

Keep your questions and directions simple.

Phrase questions so they can be answered with a "yes" or "no."

Agree on signals, such as shaking or nodding the head, or raising a hand or finger to indicate yes or no.

Use pictures, gestures, or pointing. A simple set of pictures, including a bathroom, a glass of water, food, a person walking, a person in a bed or a chair, and so on, can allow expression of needs without words (Fig. 7-15).

Use a pencil and paper if your loved one is able to write. A pencil or pen with a thick grip or with tape wrapped around it may be easier to hold.

Provide a bell or other signal so he can call you.

Common Circulatory Disorders

Hypertension or High Blood Pressure

When blood pressure consistently measures higher than 140/90, a person is diagnosed with hypertension. If blood pressure is between 120/80 and 139/89 mmHg, he or she is said to have prehypertension. This means that the person does not have high blood pressure now but is likely to have it in the future. The major cause of hypertension, or high blood pressure, is atherosclerosis, or hardening and narrowing of the blood vessels (Fig. 7-16). Hypertension can also result from kidney disease, tumors of the adrenal gland, complications of pregnancy, and head injury. Hypertension can

A	B	C	D	E	F	G	H	I	J	K	L	M
N	O	P	Q	R	S	T	U	V	W	X	Y	Z

1		2		3		4		5		6
7		8		9		10		11		12
13		14		15		16		17		18
19		20		21		22		23		24
25		26		27		28		29		30

CALL BELL	BED UP	BED DOWN	UP IN CHAIR
DOCTOR	NURSE	HUSBAND/SON	WIFE/DAUGHTER
ICE/WATER	MILK	BATHROOM	BEDPAN
RAZOR/SHAVE	GLASSES	MEDICINE	WATCH/TIME
WHEELCHAIR	BACK TO BED	TOO HOT	TOO COLD
CLERGY	HUNGRY	DRINK	TEA/COFFEE
URINAL	BRUSH TEETH	TISSUES	COMB/BRUSH
PEN/PAPER	TELEPHONE	RADIO/TV	MAGAZINE/NEWSPAPER

Fig. 7-15. A communication board can help with communication after a person has had a stroke.

develop in persons of any age.

The signs and symptoms of hypertension are not always obvious, especially in the early stages of the disease. Often the illness is only discovered when a blood pressure measurement is taken in the doctor's office. Persons with the disease may complain of headache, blurred vision, and dizziness.

Because hypertension can lead to serious conditions such as CVA, heart attack, kidney disease, and blindness, treatment to control high blood pressure is essential. If your loved one has hypertension, she may be taking medication such as cholesterol-lowering drugs and diuretics. Diuretics are drugs that reduce fluid accumulation in the body. She may also have a prescribed exercise program or be on a special low-fat, low-sodium diet. You may need to take frequent, accurate blood pressure measurements as well as encouraging her to follow her diet and exercise programs.

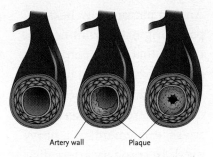

Fig. 7-16. Arteries may become hardened, or narrower, because of build-up of plaque. Hardened arteries cause high blood pressure.

Artery wall   Plaque

Coronary Artery Disease (CAD)

Coronary artery disease occurs when atherosclerosis narrows the blood vessels in the coronary arteries, reducing the supply of blood to the heart muscle and depriving it of oxygen and nutrients. Over time, as fatty deposits block the artery, the muscle that was supplied by the blood vessel dies. CAD can lead to heart attack or stroke.

Angina pectoris, or chest pain, originates from heart muscle that is not getting enough oxygen. The heart's need for oxygen is increased during exercise or exertion, stress, excitement, or a heavy meal. In coronary artery disease, constricted blood vessels prevent the extra blood with oxygen from getting to the heart (Fig. 7-17).

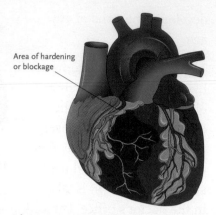

Area of hardening or blockage

Fig. 7-17. Angina pectoris results from the heart not getting enough oxygen.

The pain of angina pectoris is usually described as pressure or tightness in the left side of the chest or in the center behind the sternum or breastbone. Some people complain of pain that radiates or extends down the inside of the left arm or to the neck and left side of the jaw. A person suffering from angina pectoris may perspire or appear pale or grayish. The person may feel dizzy and have difficulty breathing.

GUIDELINES
Angina Pectoris

Rest is an extremely important aspect of care for a person who is having an episode of angina pectoris. Rest reduces the heart's need for extra oxygen, helping the blood flow return to a normal rate, often within three to fifteen minutes.

Medication is also necessary to relax the walls of the coronary arteries, allowing them to dilate, or open, to allow increased blood flow to the heart muscle. This medication, nitroglycerin, comes as a small tablet placed under the tongue, where it is

dissolved and rapidly absorbed into the circulatory system. A person who has angina pectoris should keep nitroglycerin at hand to use as soon as symptoms arise. It may also be advised that he avoid heavy meals, overeating, overexertion, and exposure to cold or hot and humid weather.

Myocardial Infarction (MI) or Heart Attack

When blood flow to the heart muscle is completely blocked, oxygen and important nutrients fail to reach the cells in that region (Fig. 7-18). Waste products are not removed and the muscle cell dies. This is called a myocardial infarction or MI, coronary thrombosis, or heart attack. The area of dead tissue may be large or small, depending on the artery involved. See chapter 13 for signs and symptoms of a myocardial infarction.

GUIDELINES
Heart Attack

Someone having a heart attack must receive emergency treatment from medical personnel to minimize damage and prevent further illness or death. Call 911 for emergency medical assistance immediately if you suspect someone is having a heart attack. Do not give him food or liquids. If you are trained to perform cardiopulmonary resuscitation (CPR), do so if necessary until help arrives.

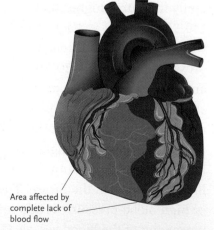

Area affected by complete lack of blood flow

Fig. 7-18. A heart attack occurs when the blood flow to the heart or a portion of the heart is cut off completely.

The care of a person recovering from a heart attack will depend on the extent of the damage, whether there have been any complications, and how long it has been since the attack occurred. In general, a person who has had a heart attack will be placed on a regular exercise program and a diet that is low in fat and cholesterol. A low-sodium diet and other changes in lifestyle may also be prescribed.

Medications may be prescribed to regulate heart rate and blood pressure.

A person recovering from a heart attack may be cautioned to avoid exposure to cold temperatures.

Congestive Heart Failure (CHF)

When heart muscle has been severely damaged by coronary artery disease, heart attack, hypertension, or other disorders, the heart fails to pump effectively. Blood backs up into the heart instead of circulating. This failure of the heart muscle to pump effectively is called congestive heart failure. It can occur on one or both sides of the heart.

Signs and symptoms of congestive heart failure include:

- difficulty breathing; coughing or gurgling with breathing
- dizziness, confusion, and fainting
- skin that appears pale or blue
- low blood pressure
- swelling of the feet and ankles
- bulging veins in the neck
- weight gain

Congestive Heart Failure

Although congestive heart failure is a serious illness, it can be successfully treated and controlled. Medications are prescribed to strengthen the heart muscle and improve its pumping action. A low-sodium diet may also be recommended. Other recommended measures include:

limited activity: a weakened heart pump may make it difficult to walk, carry groceries, or climb stairs

measurements of intake of fluids and output of urine (see chapter 12)

weight measurement to monitor accumulation of fluids (see chapter 12)

fluid reduction

low-sodium diet

application of elastic stockings to reduce swelling in feet and ankles (see chapter 11)

range of motion exercises to improve muscle tone when activity and exercise are limited (see chapter 11)

assistance with personal care and ADLs (see chapter 9)

more frequent trips to the bathroom: often those with congestive heart failure are on diuretics in addition to heart medication

observation for side effects of medications

A common side effect of medications for congestive heart failure is dizziness, which may result from a lack of potassium. This can easily be remedied by consuming high-potassium foods and drinks such as bananas, raisins, orange juice, or other citrus juices. These foods should be eaten as a preventive measure as well. Ask the doctor or pharmacist to alert you to the possible side effects of drugs and what signs or symptoms to report to the doctor.

Dementia

As we age, we typically lose some of our ability to think logically and quickly. This ability is called cognition. When we lose some of this ability we are said to have cognitive impairment. Cognitive impairment affects concentration and memory. Elderly people may lose their memories of recent events, which can be frustrating for them. You can help by encouraging them to make lists of things to remember and write down names and phone numbers.

Other normal changes of aging in the brain include slower reaction time, difficulty finding or using the right words, and sleeping less and being more wakeful at night.

Dementia is a more serious loss of mental abilities such as thinking, remembering, reasoning, and communicating. This loss makes it difficult to perform activities of daily living such as eating, bathing, dressing, and toileting. Dementia is not a normal part of aging.

The following are some of the causes of dementia:

- Alzheimer's disease

- Multi-infarct or vascular dementia (a series of strokes causing damage to the brain)

- Lewy Body disease

- Parkinson's disease

- Huntington's disease

Alzheimer's Disease

Alzheimer's disease is a progressive, degenerative, irreversible disease that causes tangled nerve fibers and protein deposits to form in the brain, eventually causing dementia. Progressive and degenerative mean the disease gets worse, causing greater and greater loss of health and abilities. Irreversible means the disease cannot be cured. Thus, a person with Alzheimer's disease will never recover and will need more and more care as the disease progresses.

As people in our society live to be older and older, more will develop Alzheimer's disease in their later years. Thus there is a growing need for care of people with Alzheimer's. Much of this care will be provided by family caregivers.

Alzheimer's disease generally begins with forgetfulness and confusion and progresses to the complete loss of all ability to care for oneself. Each person with Alzheimer's will show different symptoms at different times, so it is difficult to divide the disease into stages. For example, one person with Alzheimer's may be able to read, but may be unable to use the phone or remember her own address. Another may have lost the ability to read, but may still be able to do simple math. Skills a person has used constantly over a long lifetime are usually kept longer. Thus some people with Alzheimer's can cook or play a musical instrument with some help long after they have lost a great deal of their memory (Fig. 7-19). Look for these "preserved skills" and help your loved one use and enjoy them for as long as possible.

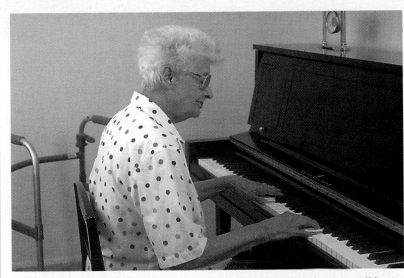

Fig. 7-19. Even when a person loses much of her memory, she may still keep skills she has used her whole life.

A person with Alzheimer's disease should be encouraged to perform activities of daily living and keep her mind and body as active as possible. Working, socializing, reading, problem solving, and exercising should all be encouraged (Fig. 7-20). Having a person with Alzheimer's do as much as possible for herself may even help slow the progression of the disease. Look for tasks that are challenging but not frustrating, and help her succeed in performing them.

It can be overwhelming to care for someone with Alzheimer's or any dementia.

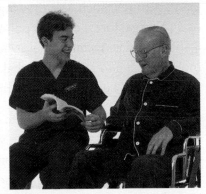

Fig. 7-20. Encourage reading and thinking activities for people with Alzheimer's disease.

It takes an enormous amount of patience, energy, dedication, and support. Certain attitudes are helpful in this challenging time:

Do not take it personally. Always remember that the person with Alzheimer's does not have control over his words and actions. He may often be unaware of what he says or does. If he doesn't recognize you, doesn't do what you say, ignores you, accuses you, or insults you, remember that it's the disease causing the behavior and not the person.

Put yourself in your loved one's shoes. Think about what it would be like to have Alzheimer's disease. Imagine being unable to bathe or feed yourself. Treat him with dignity and respect, as you would want to be treated.

Work with the symptoms and behaviors you see. Because each person with Alzheimer's disease is an individual, your loved one will not show the same symptoms as others with dementia, and may show different behaviors from day to day (Fig. 7-21). Each person with Alzheimer's will do some things that others will never do. The best strategy is to work with the behaviors you see today. For example, your loved one may want to go for a walk today, when yesterday she didn't seem able to get to the bathroom without help. If at all possible, try to take her for a walk.

Work as a team. Report your observations to the nurse,

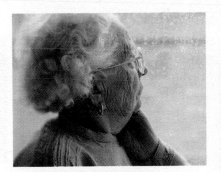

Fig. 7-21. Each person with Alzheimer's disease will not have the same symptoms at the same time. Work with the behaviors you see.

doctor, or other members of the care team. Because the symptoms and behavior of a person with Alzheimer's can change from day to day, you are in the best position to make observations about your loved one's behavior and needs.

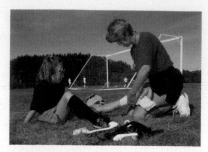

Fig. 7-22. Regular exercise is an important part of taking care of yourself.

Take care of yourself. Caring for someone with dementia can be emotionally and physically exhausting (Fig. 7-22). You need to take care of yourself in order to continue giving the best possible care.

Develop a support system. See chapter 3 for more ideas for finding resources in your community or for enlisting family and friends to help you.

Communication Strategies for Alzheimer's Disease

Speak in a low, calm voice, in a room with little background noise and distraction (Fig. 7-23). Because many people with Alzheimer's become agitated easily, it is important to do everything you can to keep them calm. This means speaking in a quiet, slow manner. It also means eliminating noise and distractions,

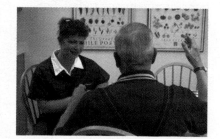

Fig. 7-23. Reduce noise and distractions when communicating with someone who has Alzheimer's disease.

such as televisions or radios, and children or others who are noisy.

Repeat yourself, using the same words and phrases, as often as needed. If your loved one does not seem to understand what you are saying or asks the same questions over and over, repeat yourself using the same words. Remember that a person with Alzheimer's literally has tangles in the brain. It may take several repetitions for a message to get through. Keep messages simple, and break complex tasks into smaller, simpler ones.

Repetition can also be reassuring for a person with Alzheimer's. In fact, many people with Alzheimer's will repeat words, phrases, questions, or actions frequently. This is called perseveration. If he perseverates, do not try to stop him. Instead, answer his questions, using the same words each time, until he stops.

Use pictures or gestures to communicate. With some people or at some point in the progression of Alzheimer's, it may be more effective to use nonverbal communication. This means using pictures, such as a drawing of a toilet on the bathroom door, and gestures, such as pointing to the closet or holding up a shirt when you want to help your loved one dress. Usually it is most effective to combine verbal and nonverbal communication, saying, "Let's get dressed now," as you hold up clothes.

Special adaptations may need to be made in the home for safety and practicality for living with Alzheimer's or any form of dementia. A nurse should visit the home and indicate changes to be made. Some of the modifications needed may include:

- Use gates on stairways (Fig. 7-24).

- Remove clutter or throw rugs.

- Use signs to mark rooms, including stop signs on rooms that should not be entered.

- Use calendars and other reminders of day, date, and location.

- Put bells on the door to indicate when someone is coming or going.

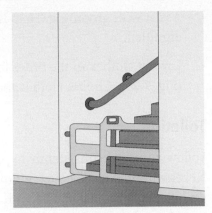

Fig. 7-24. A gate at the foot or head of the stairs will help prevent injuries. Place the gate at hip height to prevent a person from falling over it.

- Put stickers or brightly colored tape on glass doors, large windows, and glass furniture.

If your loved one wanders, you will need to take extra steps to ensure her safety:

- Put locks on doors.

- Install alarms that go off when exit doors are opened.

- Have your loved one wear identification; sew labels into clothing.

- Alert neighbors that your loved one may wander and show them a recent photo.

If your loved one paces, additional safety precautions include:

- Remove clutter and throw rugs.

- Do not rearrange furniture.

- Do not wax floors.

- Be sure that shoes and slippers fit properly and have non-slip soles.

If your loved one has difficulty walking, additional safety precautions include:

- Keep all areas of the house that your loved one uses well lit, even at night.

- Block access to stairs with a gate placed at hip height.

- Clear walkways of electrical cords.

The following are general safety tips for a person who has dementia:

- Keep medications and other chemicals out of reach.

- Display emergency numbers, including poison control, and your home address near the phone.

- Use red tape around radiators and heating vents to prevent burns.

- Check the refrigerator and any "hiding places" for spoiled food.

- Prevent kitchen accidents by removing knobs on stove, unplugging toasters and other small appliances, and supervising kitchen visits.

When your loved one's condition changes, report this to the nurse or doctor. Another visit should be made to reassess the home and make further changes as needed. For example, if she is no longer able to find the bathroom easily, signs can be posted on doors to indicate which room is which. If she begins to wander, locks can be put on all doors and labels attached to clothing to identify her if she should wander away.

If your loved one has dementia, you will probably need to provide more and more assistance as time passes. The basic procedures you use to bathe, dress, and help with eating will be described in chapter 9. The following tips are helpful when assisting the person with Alzheimer's or dementia:

- Develop a routine and stick to it. Consistency is very important when working with someone who is confused and easily agitated.

- Promote self-care. Helping your loved one to care for herself as much as possible will help her cope with this difficult disease.

- Take good care of yourself, both mentally and physically. This will help you give the best care.

More specific guidelines for assisting the person with Alzheimer's and maintaining physical and mental health are listed below.

Bathing, Grooming, and Dressing

The following suggestions can help make grooming less stressful:

- Ensure safety by using nonslip mats, tub seats, and hand holds.

- Schedule bathing when your loved one is least agitated. Be organized so the bath can be quick. Give sponge baths if he resists a shower or tub bath.

- Always use the same steps, explaining in the same way every time.

- Assist with grooming. Help him feel attractive and dignified.

- Lay out clothes in the order in which they should be put on (Fig. 7-25). Choose clothes that are simple to put on.

Toileting

Follow a routine consistently to prevent toileting problems. Never withhold or discourage fluids because a person is incontinent. Though most people with Alzheimer's will eventually experience incontinence, they may remain continent longer if these guidelines are followed:

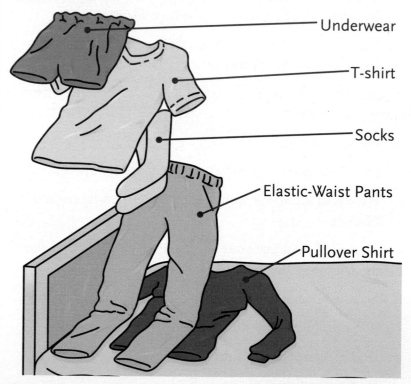

Underwear

T-shirt

Socks

Elastic-Waist Pants

Pullover Shirt

Fig. 7-25. Lay out clothes in the order in which they should be put on.

- Set up a regular schedule for toileting and follow it.

- Mark the restroom with a sign as a reminder to use it and where it is.

- Do not discourage fluids except just before bed if that is when incontinence occurs.

- Check skin regularly for signs of irritation.

- Keep track of bowel movements to avoid constipation.

Physical Health

Prevent infections by following proper procedures for food preparation and storage, household management, and using Standard Precautions. Observe the person's physical health and report any potential problems. People with dementia may not recognize their own health problems. Maintain a daily exercise routine.

Nutrition

Follow your doctor's instructions. Food may be of no interest to a person with Alzheimer's, or he may be interested in only a few types of food. In both cases, there is risk of malnutrition. Maintain optimal nutrition for a person with AD. Some ways to improve eating habits include:

- Schedule meals at the same time each day and serve familiar, appetizing foods that look and smell good.

- Provide good lighting and minimize noise and other distractions.

- If restlessness prevents getting through an entire meal, try smaller, more frequent meals. Finger foods allow eating while moving around.

- Keep the task of eating simple. Offer one course at a time using one utensil at a time. Use dishes without a pattern; white usually works best. Remove other items from the table (Fig. 7-26). Place only one item of food on the plate at a time if your loved one seems overwhelmed.

- Use adaptive equipment as needed.

- If he needs to be fed, do so slowly, offering small pieces of food. Give him time to swallow before each bite or drink.

- Do not serve steaming or very hot food or drinks.

- Encourage fluids.

- Make mealtimes simple and relaxed; allow plenty of time for eating.

- Keep nutritious snacks nearby, especially favorites.

- Observe and report changes or problems in eating habits. Monitor weight accurately and frequently to discover potential problems as soon as possible.

Mental Health

- Maintain self-esteem by encouraging self care and independence.

- Assist with personal grooming to increase self-esteem.

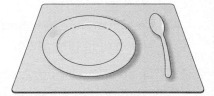

Fig. 7-26. Use white plates or bowls with a placemat in a solid color. This may help avoid confusion and distraction.

- Provide a daily calendar to encourage activities.

- Share in enjoyable activities, looking at pictures, talking, and reminiscing.

- Reward positive and independent behavior with smiles, hugs, warm touches, and thank yous.

Below are some common difficult behaviors that you may face with a person who is living with Alzheimer's. Remember that each person is different; you may or may not see these behaviors in your loved one.

1. **Agitation**. A person with dementia who is excited, restless, or troubled is said to be agitated. Situations that lead to agitation are called triggers, and may include changes in routine or caregiver, new or frustrating experiences, or even violent television. Responses that may help calm a person who is agitated include the following:

   - Try to eliminate triggers; keep routine constant.

   - Avoid frustration.

   - Focus on a soothing, familiar activity, such as sorting things or looking at pictures.

   - Remain calm and use a low, soothing voice to speak to and reassure her.

   - An arm around the shoulder, patting, or stroking may be soothing (Fig. 7-27).

2. **Pacing and Wandering**. A person with dementia who walks back and forth in the same area is pacing. Someone who walks aimlessly around the house or neighborhood is wandering. Pacing and wandering may have some of the following causes:

- restlessness

- hunger

- disorientation

- need for toileting

- forgetting how or where to sit down

- too much daytime napping

- need for exercise

- pain

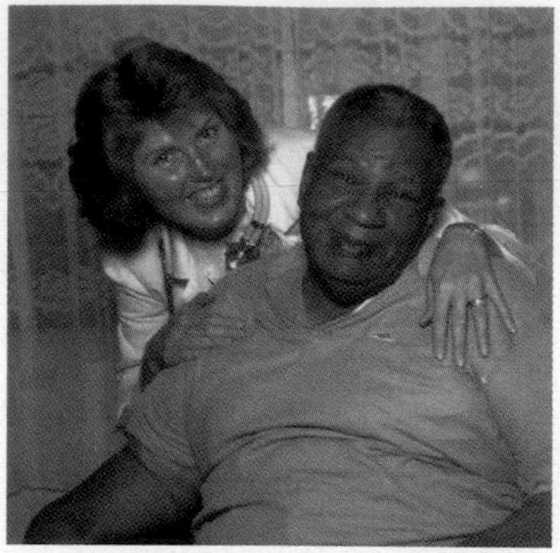

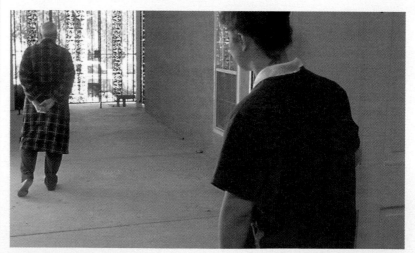

Fig. 7-27. Warm touches and hugs may soothe someone with Alzheimer's disease.

Responses to pacing and wandering include the following:

- Let your loved one pace or wander in a safe and secure (locked) area where you can watch him, such as in a level, fenced yard (Fig. 7-28).

Fig. 7-28. Make sure your loved one is in a safe area if he paces or wanders.

- Eliminate causes when you can: for example, provide nutritious snacks, encourage an exercise routine, and maintain a toileting schedule.

- Suggest another activity, such as going for a walk together.

3. **Hallucinations or Delusions**. A person with dementia who sees things that are not there is having hallucinations (Fig. 7-29). Someone who believes things that are not true is having delusions (Fig. 7-30). You can respond to hallucinations or delusions in the following ways:

   - Ignore harmless hallucinations and delusions.

   - Reassure her if she seems agitated or worried.

   - Do not argue with a person who is imagining things. Remember that the feelings are real to her. Redirect her to other activities or thoughts.

   - Be calm and reassure her that you are there to help.

4. **Sundowning**. When a person becomes restless and agitated in the late afternoon, evening, or night, it is called sundowning. Sundowning may be triggered by hunger, fatigue, a change in routine or caregiver, or any new or frustrating situation. These are some effective responses to sundowning:

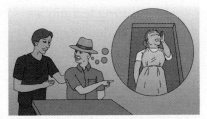

Fig. 7-29. Hallucinating is seeing or hearing things that are not really there. For example, a person thinks he hears his aunt calling him to dinner. You know that his aunt died twenty years ago, but to him this is very real.

   - Eliminate triggers by providing snacks or encouraging rest.

- Avoid stressful situations during this time; limit activities, appointments, trips, and visits.

- Play soft music.

- Set a bedtime routine and keep it.

- Recognize when sundowning occurs and plan a calming activity just before this time.

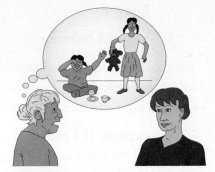

Fig. 7-30. A delusion is a belief in something that is not true, or is out of touch with reality. For example, a person thinks that her long-deceased sister is taking things from her, like she did when they were young.

- Eliminate caffeine from the diet.

- Give a soothing back massage.

- Redirect the behavior or distract with a simple, calm activity like looking at a magazine.

- Maintain a daily exercise routine.

5. **Catastrophic Reactions**. When a person with Alzheimer's overreacts to something in an unreasonable way, it is called a catastrophic reaction. It may be triggered by any of the following:

   - fatigue

   - change of routine, environment, or caregiver

   - overstimulation: too much noise or activity

   - difficult choices or tasks

   - physical pain

Meeting Special Needs and Conditions

7

- hunger
- need for toileting

You can respond to catastrophic reactions as you would to agitation or sundowning. For example, eliminate triggers and try to focus on a soothing activity.

6. **Depression**. If a person becomes withdrawn, has no energy, does not want to eat or do things he used to enjoy, he may be depressed (Fig. 7-31). Depression may have many causes, including:

- loss of independence
- inability to cope
- feelings of failure, fear
- facing a progressive, degenerative illness

You can respond to depression in a number of ways:

- Report signs of depression to your doctor. It is an illness that can be treated with medication.

- Encourage independence, self-care, and activity.

- Talk about moods and feelings if your loved one is willing. Be a good listener.

- Encourage social interaction.

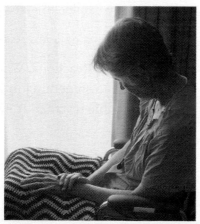

Fig. 7-31. A person who is withdrawn and has no energy may be depressed. It is very important to report signs of depression to the doctor.

7. **Perseveration or Repetitive Phrasing**. A person who repeats a word, phrase, question, or activity over and over is perseverating. Repeating a word or phrase is also called repetitive phrasing. Such behavior may be caused by several factors, including disorientation or confusion. Respond to perseveration with patience. Do not try to silence or stop your loved one. Answer questions each time they are asked, using the same words each time.

8. **Violent Behavior**. A person who attacks, hits, or threatens someone is violent. Violence may be triggered by many situations, including frustration, overstimulation, or a change in routine, environment, or caregiver.

The following are appropriate responses to violent behavior:

- Block blows but never hit back (Fig. 7-32).
- Step out of reach.
- Call for help if needed.
- Do not leave the person in the home alone.
- Try to eliminate triggers.
- Use calming techniques as you would for agitation or sundowning.

Although Alzheimer's is an irreversible disease, meaning it cannot be cured, there are many techniques that can improve the quality of life for people with Alzheimer's. Some are described below.

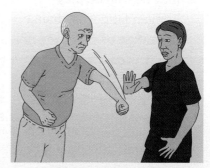

Fig. 7-32. Block blows but do not hit back.

Reality orientation is the use of calendars, clocks, signs, and lists to reorient your loved one and help her remember who and where she is. It is most useful in the early stages of Alzheimer's, when a person is confused but not totally disoriented. In later stages, reality orientation may only be frustrating.

Example: Each day, you show your mother the calendar and point out what day of the week it is. On the calendar or another piece of paper, you list all the things you will do that day; for example, take a bath, go for a walk, eat lunch, and play cards. Whenever you speak to her, you call her "Mother," as you always have. When helping her with tasks, explain why you do things as you do. For example, "We use a tub seat in the shower so you don't have to stand up for so long, Mother."

Benefits: Using the calendar, making lists, and using names frequently help your loved one stay in touch with the world around her. This will help her feel more in control of her life. It will also allow her to do as much as possible for herself. Explaining what you do and why you do it as you assist her will make her feel more like a participant in her care and less like an invalid.

Validation therapy is letting a person believe he lives in the past or in imaginary circumstances by exploring and validating his beliefs. Validating means giving value to or approving, and making no attempt to reorient him to actual circumstances. It is useful in cases of moderate to severe disorientation.

Example: Your uncle tells you he does not want to eat lunch today because he is going out to a restaurant later with his wife. Your aunt has been dead for many years and Uncle Paul can no longer eat out in restaurants. Instead of telling him that he is not going out to eat, you ask what restaurant he is going to, what he will have, and what time he is going. You suggest that he eat a good lunch now because sometimes the service is slow in restaurants and he might get hungry while waiting.

Benefits: By "playing along" with Uncle Paul's fantasy, you let him know that you take him seriously. You do not think of him as a crazy person or a child who does not know what is happening in his own life.

Reminiscence therapy is encouraging someone to reminisce, to remember and talk about the past (Fig. 7-33). Explore his memories by asking about details. Focus on a time of life that was more pleasant for him, or work through feelings about a difficult time in the past. It is useful in many stages of Alzheimer's, but especially with moderate to severe confusion.

Example: Your father-in-law, a 77-year-old man with Alzheimer's, fought in World War II. In his home are many

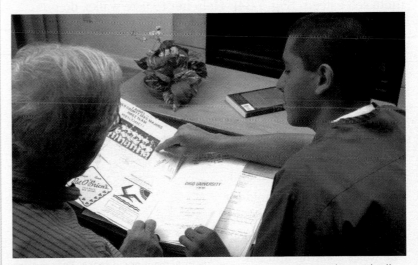

Fig. 7-33. Reminiscence therapy encourages a person to remember and talk about his past.

mementos of the war: pictures of his war buddies, a medal he was given, and more. You ask him to tell you where he was sent in the war, and he tells you a little bit about being in the Pacific. You ask him more detailed questions about his experiences, and eventually he tells you about many things: the friends he made in the service, why he was given the medal, times when he was scared and how much he missed his wife and children.

Benefits: By asking questions about your father-in-law's experiences in the war, you remind him that he was once a person who was competent, social, responsible, and brave. This boosts his self-esteem. Even though you may have heard these stories many times before, listening shows your respect and creates a positive atmosphere in the home.

Activity therapy involves using activities, especially those your loved one enjoys, to prevent boredom and frustration and promote self-esteem (Fig. 7-34). Help her to take walks, do puzzles, listen to music, cook, read, or do other activities she enjoys. It is useful throughout most stages of Alzheimer's, depending on the activity.

Example: Your grandmother, a 70-year-old woman with Alzheimer's, raised four children and ran a household for almost 50 years before being diagnosed with Alzheimer's. She loves cooking and baking and misses being in the

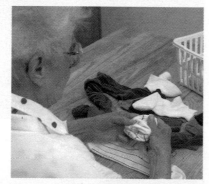

Fig. 7-34. Activities that are not frustrating can be helpful for a person with Alzheimer's disease. They promote mental exercise.

kitchen now that she cannot cook for herself. Nana always used to bake cookies at Christmas for the whole family, and you know she would love to be able to bake cookies this year. You purchase some pre-made cookie dough and roll it out. Nana uses her old cookie cutters to cut out the shapes. You bake the cookies for her, and another day she can decorate them.

Benefits: Nana can enjoy an activity that always brought her pleasure. She feels competent, because you gave her small tasks, such as cutting out the cookies, that she could handle.

Chronic Obstructive Pulmonary Disease (COPD)

People diagnosed with COPD are often ill for a long time. Because it is a chronic disease, a person with COPD may live for years but never be cured. Those with COPD have difficulty breathing, especially expelling air from the lungs. There are four different chronic lung diseases that are categorized under COPD; they are chronic bronchitis, pulmonary emphysema, asthma, and chronic bronchiectstasis.

Over time, a person with any of these lung disorders becomes weakened and is at high risk for acute infections of the lungs, such as pneumonia. When the lungs and brain do not get enough oxygen, all the body systems are affected. People with COPD may live in constant fear of not being able to breathe. Sometimes this causes them to remain upright in an attempt to improve their ability to expand the lungs. They often have poor appetites. They usually do not get adequate sleep. These factors can add to overall weakness and poor health. There is a great sense of loss of control over the body with COPD, particularly with breathing. Agitation and fear of suffocation may be present.

A person who is living with COPD may experience the following symptoms:

- Chronic cough or wheeze

- Difficulty breathing, especially when breathing deeply

- Shortness of breath, especially during exercise or activity

- Pale, cyanotic (bluish), or reddish-purple skin color

- Mental confusion

- General state of weakness

- Fear and anxiety

GUIDELINES
COPD

Observe for worsening of symptoms and report them promptly to the doctor.

Encourage your loved one to find a comfortable sitting position. Provide pillows for support. An upright, forward-leaning body position is recommended (Fig. 7-35).

Offer plenty of fluids and frequent meals.

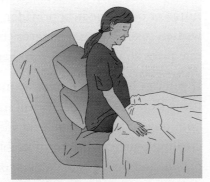

Fig. 7-35. It helps people with COPD to sit upright and lean forward slightly.

Encourage good nutrition and a well-balanced diet.

Keep and use oxygen as ordered by the doctor (see chapter 11).

Try to maintain a calm and supportive environment.

Use good infection control procedures (see chapter 5), especially handwashing and proper disposal of used tissues.

Encourage independence and self-care.

Try to avoid situations in which your loved one may be exposed to infections, especially colds or flu. Discourage visits from anyone who is unwell. Ask all visitors to wash their hands when they arrive.

Have an emergency plan in case of a breathing crisis. Your doctor should instruct you as to what measures to take.

Teach pursed-lip breathing. Place the lips as if in a kiss and take controlled breaths.

Keep the home free of hazards.

Encourage your loved one to save energy for important daily tasks and to rest as needed during tasks.

Hip or Knee Replacement

These surgeries have become more common in recent years. Depending on the reason for the surgery and the person's age, recuperation can be quite extensive. The surgeon and the physical therapist will give you specific instructions about caring for someone after this type of surgery. The general discussion and guidelines for care below are intended only to supplement those instructions.

Meeting Special Needs and Conditions

7

Total hip replacement is surgery performed to replace the head of the long bone of the leg (femur) at the joint where it meets the hip. This may be performed due to a fracture caused by an injury, weakness caused by age, or pain caused by loss of bone strength.

The surgery is done through an incision at the hip, where an artificial ball and socket joint replaces the poorly functioning or damaged hip. After the surgery, the person is not able to bear weight on that leg while the area heals. The goals for rehabilitation generally include strengthening the hip muscles so the person can walk on the affected leg again.

Follow instructions carefully regarding when your loved one can bear weight on the new hip and how much she can do. She will need help with personal care, and she will need to use canes or walkers as ordered by the doctor or physical therapist.

GUIDELINES
Hip Replacement

Keep often used items, such as medications, telephone, tissues and water, in easy reach. Avoid placing items in high places.

Dress the affected, or weaker, side first.

Never rush. Praise and encourage even small accomplishments.

Have her sit to do tasks when possible to save energy.

The hip cannot be bent more than 90 degrees or turned inward. A person recovering from hip replacement surgery should not cross his legs (Fig. 7-36).

Total knee replacement is the surgical insertion of a hinged prosthesis as a new joint. This is done to relieve pain and re-store motion to a knee damaged by injury or arthritis. Recovery time should be shorter than for hip replacement, but care guidelines are similar.

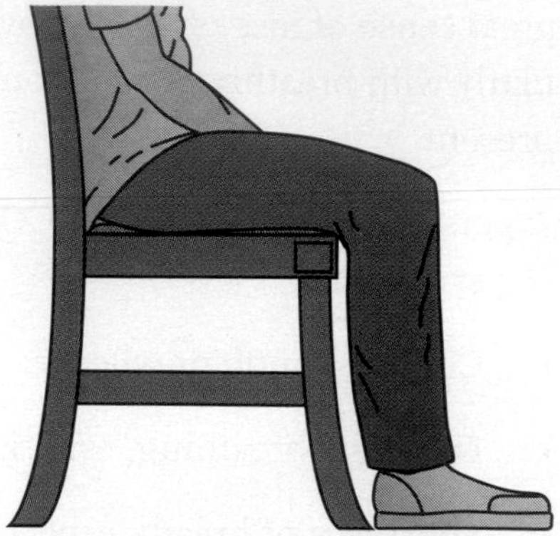

Fig. 7-36. The hip must maintain a 90-degree angle in the sitting position.

GUIDELINES
Knee Replacement

Special stockings, such as compression stockings or anti-embolic stockings, can be applied to prevent blood clots.

Encourage fluids, especially cranberry and orange juice, which contain Vitamin C, to prevent urinary tract infections.

Depending on the type of surgery, you may need to make extensive adaptations for your loved one's homecoming. Try to learn as much as you can before he is discharged from the hospital, and be sure you know whom to call with questions after you are home. If it is possible to have a home visit from a nurse or other medical provider, take advantage of it. Ask for written instructions whenever you can, and keep all papers in one place so you can refer to them later.

If you can have the home organized before your loved one returns from the hospital, it will make the transition easier on both of you. See chapter 4 for ideas on removing hazards and creating practical and comfortable spaces for the recuperating person and for visitors. When someone offers to help, suggest that a prepared meal ready to serve when you come home would be helpful and comforting.

Resources

The Arthritis Foundation site has information and links to resources for those with arthritis, including a link to find your local chapter. There is a buyer's guide for products that are easy for people with arthritis to use, and a link for contacting your congressperson about issues relating to arthritis.

Arthritis Foundation
PO Box 7669
Atlanta, GA 30357-0669
Tel: 800-283-7800
www.arthritis.org

The American Cancer Society site contains information for those who have cancer and their families and friends, as well as support resources for survivors of cancer and tips for prevention and early detection. There is a locator that you can use to find activities and resources in your community.

American Cancer Society
Tel: 800-ACS-2345
www.cancer.org

The United Ostomy Association's website offers information for people of various age groups who have had diversionary surgery. There is also information about prevention of and screening for colon cancer and updates of relevant medical news.

United Ostomy Association, Inc.
19772 MacArthur Blvd., #200
Irvine, CA 92612-2405
Tel: 800-826-0826
www.uoa.org

The American Diabetes Association's website includes news and information about diabetes, including research and prevention. There is information about nutrition, including recipes, and information especially for parents and children.

American Diabetes Association
1701 North Beauregard Street
Alexandria, VA 22311
Tel: 800-DIABETES (800-342-2383)
www.diabetes.org

SAFE is an international Internet coalition of stroke survivors, their loved ones, and healthcare professionals who work in the field. The site has information about stroke and signs of stroke as well as links to support resources.

SAFE (Stroke Awareness for Everyone)
8906 E. 96th St., #311
Fishers, IN 46038
Fax: 317-585-9563
www.strokesafe.org

The Stroke Information Directory contains information about stroke and therapy for those recovering from stroke as well as a locator for regional facilities that treat stroke.

Stroke Information Directory (SID)
E-mail: ndk@stroke-info.com
www.stroke-info.com

The Pulmonary Hypertension Association addresses pulmonary hypertension, or continuous high blood pressure in the lungs, which can lead to an enlarged heart. The site contains health information, *links to support resources and a special section with insurance information.*

Pulmonary Hypertension Association (PHA)
850 Sligo Avenue, Suite 800
Silver Spring, MD 20910
Tel: 800-748-7274
www.phassociation.org

The American Heart Association offers information on heart health and heart diseases and conditions. Their site provides a link that allows you to find your local AHA branch.

American Heart Association
National Center
7272 Greenville Avenue
Dallas, TX 75231
Tel: 800-AHA-USA-1 or 800-242-8721
www.americanheart.org

The National Heart, Lung, and Blood Institute's website is sponsored by the Department of Health and Human Services and the National Institutes for Health. It has sections for patients and their families, health care professionals, and researchers. The section for patients is focused on education; there is also a link to a list of clinical trials.

National Heart, Lung, and Blood Institute
PO Box 30105
Bethesda, MD 20824-0105
Tel: 301-592-8573
www.nhlbi.nih.gov

The HeartCenterOnline's site is focused on providing users with the tools they need to educate themselves and monitor their own health. The site also provides links to information about other health topics such as cancer, women's health, and mental health.

HeartCenterOnline (part of HealthCentersOnline)
One South Ocean Boulevard, Suite 201
Boca Raton, FL 33432
Fax: 561-620-9799
www.heartcenteronline.com

The Alzheimer's Disease Education and Referral Center provides current, comprehensive Alzheimer's disease (AD) information and resources from the U.S. Government's National Institute on Aging (NIA).

Alzheimer's Disease Education and Referral Center (a service of the National Institute on Aging)
ADEAR Center
PO Box 8250
Silver Spring, MD 20907-8250
Tel: 800-438-4380
www.alzheimers.org

The Alzheimer's Association provides information about AD as well as articles concerning the latest research in the field. There is also an advocacy link for those who would like to take an active role in fighting Alzheimer's disease.

Alzheimer's Association
225 N. Michigan Ave. Fl. 17
Chicago, IL 60601-7633
Tel: 800-272-3900
www.alz.org

The COPD International's website has information for those with COPD and their caregivers as well as information for kids and teens. There are tips for coping, links to support resources both on-line and offline, and detailed information on the latest drugs being used to treat COPD.

COPD International
131 D.W. Highway #627
Nashua, NH 03060
www.copd-international.com

The American Lung Association's website has information on various lung diseases, including cancer and COPD. There are comprehensive descriptions of treatment options for these diseases and interactive tools to help users better understand their own condition and options. The site has a great deal of support information, including support for those who are trying to quit smoking.

The American Lung Association
61 Broadway, 6th Floor
NY, NY 10006
Tel: 800-LUNGUSA
www.lungusa.org

8

Death, Dying, and Hospice Care

If your loved one is elderly or has a terminal disease, you will eventually face the issues of dying and death. The purpose of this chapter is to provide information that may help you think about these issues both before and at the time of death. As you have probably already discovered, caregiving involves far more than the physical tasks of keeping house and driving your loved one to the doctor, as demanding as these may be. As a caregiver, you provide not only physical care but also emotional support (Fig. 8-1). The end of life can be the time when emotional demands on you become the most intense.

It may never be possible to prepare oneself emotionally for the death of a loved one, but many have found that familiarity with the stages of death and the processes of grief can be helpful at this difficult time. As always in caregiving, do not try to go it alone. You need support now more than ever. Find some-

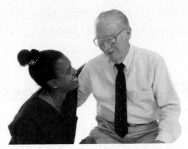

Fig. 8-1. As a caregiver, you provide emotional support as well as physical care.

one who will listen, comfort you, give you a break, or put things into perspective for you. One of the positive elements of hospice care is the support its employees can offer to families and friends of the person who is dying or who has died.

First Steps

If your loved one has a terminal illness, the first thing to do is get as much information as you can about her needs and wishes. Find out from her physician what the likely progression of the disease will be—what symptoms will occur, how they can be treated, and how best to make her as comfortable as possible while allowing her to retain as much independence and dignity as possible.

Find out from your loved one what her wishes are. Does she have, or wish to create, any advance directives? More information on advance directives is found in chapter 1. What are her wishes regarding ceremonies and burial after her death? Read

"The Dying Person's Bill of Rights" in this chapter, and decide together with your loved one how best to preserve her rights. Once you have made yourself aware of your loved one's wishes, seek out a physician or organization that can help to meet them. Use the resources at the end of this chapter, or ask your loved one's physician or another trusted healthcare provider for help.

Seek support for yourself during this difficult time. Talk to friends, clergy, a therapist or a member of the healthcare team about your fears and feelings.

The Stages of Dying

Death can occur suddenly and without warning, or it can be expected. Older people or those with terminal illnesses may have time to prepare for death. Preparing for death is a process that involves the dying person's emotions and behavior.

Dr. Elisabeth Kubler-Ross researched and wrote about the process of dying. Her book, *On Death and Dying*, describes five stages that dying people and their families or friends may experience before death. These five stages are described below. Not everyone will go through all the stages. Some may stay in one stage until death occurs. Some may move back and forth between stages during the process.

Denial. A person in the denial stage may refuse to believe she is dying. She may believe that a mistake has been made. She may talk about the future and avoid any discussion of her illness. This stage may last a few hours, days, or longer. Some people are still in the denial stage at the time of death. This is the "No. Not me." stage.

Anger. Once she starts to face the possibility of her death, a person with terminal illness will usually become angry that she is dying. She may be angry because she believes she is too young or because she has always been "good" or taken care of herself. She is not yet ready to accept the idea of her death. Anger is a normal and healthy reaction. Try not to take this anger personally. This is the "Why me?" stage.

Bargaining. Once a person has begun to believe that she really is dying, she may make promises to God or somehow try to bargain for her recovery. She may promise to do something special or change her life if she is allowed to recover or live longer. This is the "Yes me, but..." stage.

Depression. As she becomes physically weaker and symptoms of the progressing illness become more pronounced, a person who is dying may become deeply sad or depressed (Fig. 8-2). She mourns for her life and may talk about all the things she is leaving behind. She may cry or withdraw into silence or be unable to perform even simple activities. She needs physical and emotional support both from you and from skilled healthcare providers. At this stage, she will need to be able to review her life and her feelings. It is important to listen and be understanding at this stage.

Acceptance. Sometimes the person who is dying is eventually able to accept death and prepare for it. She may make plans for her last days

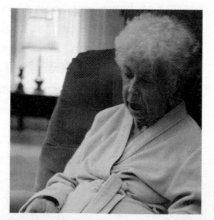

Fig. 8-2. A person who is dying may become depressed.

or for the ceremonies that may follow. At this stage, she may seem emotionally detached.

The Grief Process

Just as dying is a process with different stages, dealing with grief after the death of a loved one is a process as well. We may find ourselves experiencing several feelings at once or passing through different stages of grief at different times. As with dying, grieving is an individual process; no two people will grieve in exactly the same way. Clergy, counselors, or social workers can provide help for people who are grieving (Fig, 8-3). You may have any of the following reactions to the death of a loved one:

Shock. Even when death was expected, we may still be shocked when death occurs. Many of us do not know what to expect after the death of a loved one. We may be surprised by our feelings, even when we knew death was coming.

Denial. Sometimes we want to believe that everything will quickly return to normal after a death. We want to believe that we do not have many feelings to cope with.

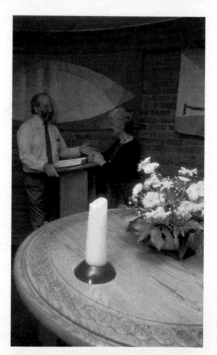

Fig. 8-3. Clergy may provide comfort for those who are grieving.

Denying or refusing to acknowledge grief can help people deal with the first hours or days after a death. But eventually we must face our feelings. Grief can be so overwhelming for some people that they may take years to face their feelings. Professional help can be very valuable at such a time.

Anger. Although it is hard to admit it, many of us feel angry after a death. We may be angry at ourselves, at God, at the doctors, or even at the person who died. There is nothing wrong with feeling anger as part of grief.

Guilt. It is very common for families, friends, and even unrelated caregivers to feel guilty after a death. We may wish we had done more for our loved one, or we may simply feel that he did not deserve to die any more than we do. We may feel guilty that we are still living.

Regret. Often after a death we have regrets about what we did or did not do for our loved one. We may regret things we said or did not say. Many people carry these regrets with them for years.

Sadness. Feeling depressed or down is very common after a death. We may cry or feel emotionally unstable. We may suffer headaches or insomnia when we cannot express our sadness.

Loneliness. Missing someone who has died is very normal and can bring up other feelings, such as sadness or regret. Many things may remind us of our loved one who has died. The memories may be painful at first. With time, we usually feel less lonely and memories become more positive and less painful.

Do not be afraid to seek support in dealing with your grief after the death of a loved one. Particularly when you have been a caregiver, death causes dramatic change in your daily life which can make grief seem even more overwhelming. You may not know what to do with yourself now that your life is no longer filled up with the daily tasks of caregiving and all the busy urgency is replaced by feelings of sadness, regret, and loneliness. There are many support groups and other resources for those who are grieving. Look for these through hospice agencies, hospitals, churches or synagogues (Fig 8-4).

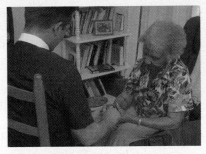

Fig. 8-4. Talking can help healing after the death of a loved one.

Signs of Approaching Death

Death can be sudden or gradual. Certain physical changes occur that can be recognized as signs and symptoms of approaching death. Changes occur in the circulatory system that affect the vital signs and skin color. The central nervous system shows signs of deterioration that may include disorientation, confusion, and reduced reflexes and responsiveness. Vision, taste, and touch usually diminish; however, hearing is often present until death occurs. Signs of approaching death include:

- blurred and failing vision

- unfocused eyes

- impaired speech

- diminished sense of touch

- loss of movement, muscle tone, and feeling

- a rising or below-normal body temperature

- decreasing blood pressure

- weak pulse that is abnormally slow or rapid

- slow, irregular respirations or rapid, shallow respirations, called Cheyne-Stokes respirations

- a "rattling" or "gurgling" sound as the person breathes

- cold, pale skin

- mottling, spotting, or blotching of the skin caused by poor circulation

- perspiration

- incontinence (both urine and stool)

- disorientation or confusion

Providing Care at the Time of Death

Most people who have been present at a number of deaths believe it is calmer and more comfortable for a person to die at home (Fig. 8-5). If you are present as your loved one dies, you may find yourself dealing with many emotions as well as many physical tasks. As difficult as it may be for you, your presence is probably deeply reassuring to your loved one. Remember this, and know that there are several things you can do to help her feel more comfortable.

I have the right to:

be treated as a living human being until I die.

maintain a sense of hopefulness, however changing its focus may be.

be cared for by those who can maintain a sense of hopefulness, however changing this might be.

express my feelings and emotions about my approaching death in my own way.

participate in decisions concerning my care.

expect continuing medical and nursing attention even though "cure" goals must be changed to "comfort" goals.

to die alone.

be free from pain.

have my questions answered honestly.

not be deceived.

have help from and for my family in accepting my death.

die in peace and dignity.

retain my individuality and not be judged for my decisions which may be contrary to the beliefs of others.

discuss and enlarge my religious and/or spiritual experiences, whatever these may mean to others.

expect that the sanctity of the human body will be respected after death.

be cared for by caring, sensitive, knowledgeable people who will attempt to understand my needs and will be able to gain some satisfaction in helping me face my death.

Fig. 8-5. The Dying Person's Bill of Rights. (This was created at a workshop on "The Terminally Ill Patient and the Helping Person," sponsored by Southwestern Michigan In-Service Education Council, and appeared in the *American Journal of Nursing*, Vol. 75, January 1975, p.99.

GUIDELINES
Caring for a Dying Person

Diminished Senses. As vision fails the dying person, she naturally turns toward light. She may fear the dark. Keep the room softly lit and without glare. Because she cannot see well but may still be able to hear, tell her about any procedures that are being done or anything that is happening in the room.

Speaking may become difficult for your loved one, but hearing usually remains until death occurs. Therefore, talk in a normal voice but do not expect an answer. Ask few questions and only those that require a simple yes or no answer. Avoid subjects that are disturbing. Anticipate your loved one's needs by observing body language.

Eating and Drinking. Food becomes difficult to swallow and digest. As eating and drinking decreases, offer ice chips, cold liquids, and gelatin, ice cream, or frozen yogurt.

Care of the Eyes, Nose, and Mouth. Mucous secretions in the eyes, nose, and mouth may collect and become uncomfortable. As your loved one drinks less fluids and his mouth becomes dry, you will need to provide mouth care frequently. The skin around his eyes can be bathed with normal saline solution. A lubricant may be applied lightly to the lips and nose if irritation and crusting occur.

Changes in Breathing. Breathing may become irregular with progressively longer periods of no breathing. The person may seem to be sucking air or working very hard to breathe. Mucus may collect in the back of the throat and may rattle or gurgle as the person breathes through his mouth. Raising the person's head, raising the head of the bed, or turning him on his side may help (Fig. 8-6). A cool room and a fan may also help if your loved one has a history of respiratory problems.

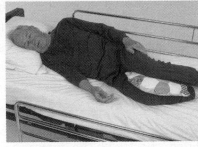

Fig. 8-6. Turning a person on his side may help alleviate breathing problems. Pillows help provide extra support.

Skin Care. If your loved one is perspiring, bathe her as needed and change her sheets and clothes for her comfort. Skin care to prevent pressure sores is still important in the last days of life, especially for someone who is immobile or incontinent. Keep sheets wrinkle-free. Waterproof pads or disposable pads may be used, or a catheter may be placed to manage urine. She should be kept clean and dry.

Comfort. Pain relief is very important (Fig. 8-7). Your loved one may not be able to communicate that he is in pain; observe him for signs of pain and report them. Make him comfortable with frequent changes of position, back massage, good skin care, frequent mouth care, and proper body alignment. This type of care is discussed more in chapter 9. Because body temperature usually increases, he may be more comfortable with light covers, even when his skin feels cool to the touch. He may perspire more.

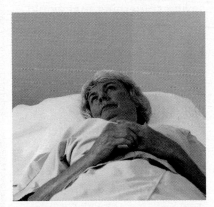

Fig. 8-7. Pain relief is very important; be alert for signs that your loved one is in pain.

Restlessness or Mental Confusion. A person who is dying may become agitated or confused. He may pick at the bed linens or try to get out of bed. This occurs due to decreased oxygen to the brain, failure of the kidneys to function, or dreams and hallucinations. If restlessness occurs, speak to your loved one in a calm and normal tone of voice while touching him softly or holding his hand. If he becomes combative or extremely agitated, check with the doctor to see if medication is needed.

Environment. Display favorite objects, photographs, cards, flowers, religious items, and mementos in places where your loved one can easily see them. These can provide comfort. Cover medical equipment that may be disturbing. Make sure the room is comfortable, appropriately lit, and well ventilated (Fig. 8-8).

Emotional and Spiritual Support. We often feel uncomfortable talking with those who are seriously ill or who are dying. We are afraid of saying something that would be upsetting or inappropriate. What most people who are dying need, however, is not words. In the early stages of death, they may need someone who will listen to them as they reflect on their lives or discuss their fears and concerns about dying. Later on they may simply need the quiet, reassuring, and loving presence of another person.

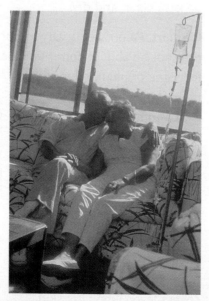

Fig. 8-8. Provide as comfortable an environment as possible for your loved one.

Touch can be very important. Holding your loved one's hand as you sit quietly can be very comforting. A person who is dying may also seek spiritual comfort from clergy members.

Postmortem Care

Postmortem care means care of the body after death. Depending on who is present at the time of death and where the body is to be taken, postmortem care may be performed in the home by a nurse, an aide, or other provider. Postmortem care usually includes the following steps:

GUIDELINES
Postmortem Care

Bathe the body. Be gentle to avoid bruising. Place drainage pads where needed, most often under the head and/or under the perineum. Be sure to follow Standard Precautions.

Decide how the person will be dressed.

Do not remove any tubes or other equipment. A nurse will do this, or the funeral home will do it later.

Insert dentures and close the mouth. You may need to place a rolled towel under the chin to support the closed mouth position.

Close the eyes carefully.

Position the body on the back, with legs straight, arms folded across the abdomen, and a small pillow under the head.

Strip the bed after the body has been removed.

Open windows, as appropriate, and straighten up the room.

Arrange personal items carefully so they are not lost.

Hospice Care

Hospice is a compassionate method of caring for people with a terminal illness and their families. Hospice care uses a holistic approach, treating the whole person, including physical, emotional, spiritual, and social needs. Hospice care can be provided 24 hours a day, seven days a week. Hospice care may be provided in a hospital, a special hospice facility, or in the home. A hospice can be any location where a person who is dying is treated with dignity by caregivers who are specially trained to holistically provide for the needs of the dying person and her loved ones.

In hospice care, the goals of care are the comfort and dignity of the person rather than his recovery. Hospice caregivers have a different mindset than other healthcare providers; they focus on relieving pain and making the person comfortable.

Besides pain relief, comfort, personal care, and emotional and spiritual support, a person who is dying also needs to feel some independence for as long as possible. Try to let your loved one retain as much control over her life as possible. Eventually, though, you or someone else may have to meet all of her basic needs.

Hospice care may be provided by any caregiver, but often specially trained nurses, social workers, and volunteers participate in hospice care. The hospice team may also include physicians, counselors, home health aides, therapists, clergy, and dietitians.

According to the National Hospice and Palliative Care Organization, there are now 3,300 hospices across the country. They gave care to more than 950,000 people in 2003. About 400,000 hospice volunteers give more than 18 million hours each year to help people who are dying.

Hospice workers are trained to offer support not only to the person who is dying, but to the family and friends who will survive and mourn. Some of the services that they provide include caring for the home and family of a dying person, driving or doing errands, and emotional support. Hospice can be an excellent place for you to turn for support before, during, and after the death of your loved one.

Resources

The National Hospice and Palliative Care Organization provides information and answers questions about hospice care. There is a database in which you can search for hospice and palliative care organizations in your area.

National Hospice and Palliative Care Organization (NHPCO)
1700 Diagonal Road, Suite 625
Alexandria, Virginia 22314
Tel: 703-837-1500
Fax: 703-837-1233
www.nho.org

The Hospice Foundation of America provides support to those who are dealing with terminal illness, death and the grief and bereavement process, including medical professionals and volunteers. There is a link to a locator service that can help you find hospice care available in your area.

Hospice Foundation of America
Tel: 800-854-3402
www.hospicefoundation.org

The U.S. Living Will Registry provides information about advance directives and links to advance directive forms for each state. As discussed in chapter 1, advance directives are documents that allow people to choose what kind of medical care they wish to have in the event they are unable to make those decisions themselves. An advance directive can also designate someone else to make medical decisions for a person if that person is incapacitated. Living Wills and Durable Power of Attorney for Health Care are examples of advance directives.

U.S. Living Will Registry
523 Westfield Ave., PO Box 2789
Westfield, NJ 07091-2789
Tel: 800-LIV-WILL (800-548-9455)
Fax: 908-654-1919
www.uslivingwillregistry.com

Federal law requires all hospitals to provide information about advance directives to people in their communities, including information about the laws specific to that state.

9

Providing Personal Care

If your loved one is ill, he may not have the energy to care for himself. He may need help with personal care; he may even need you to provide it for him entirely. This chapter will show you how to help with personal care while still helping him maintain independence and dignity.

First Steps

Consult a healthcare professional, such as a physician, registered nurse, or a physical or occupational therapist to learn if procedures in this book are appropriate for your loved one. If they are appropriate, have the professional show you how to perform each procedure, including adaptations for your loved one. Make sure that you are competent and comfortable doing any procedure before attempting it on your own.

Make sure to obtain enough of all of the personal care supplies that you will need for each procedure you will be performing. Be sure to monitor supplies closely so that you will not run out of anything you need.

Make sure that you are strong enough to perform the procedures that require lifting or weight bearing, such as assisting with transfers. Be sure to obtain any assistive devices necessary, especially if you are not absolutely certain that someone will always be available to assist you. Make yourself aware of good body mechanics to reduce the likelihood of injury to yourself and your loved one.

It is a good idea to discuss each of these personal care procedures with your loved one before it becomes necessary to perform them. This way you can be sure that you know her preferences and expectations and she will know exactly how things will be done.

When home health aides are trained to provide care, the heart of their training is the procedures they are taught to perform. These include everything from handwashing to taking a client's temperature, helping a client transfer from a bed to a chair, and helping a client to use a bedpan. There is an established, medically accepted way to perform each of these activities. Home health aides are trained, tested, and certified according to very specific guidelines.

Much of the material in this book was originally developed to train certified home health aides; thus, many of the photographs show uniformed professionals providing care. This information has been used in thousands of successful training programs; it is regularly reviewed and updated to meet the latest medical standards. If your loved one receives care from a home health aide, you will see some of these procedures performed in your home. You may wish to know the accepted procedures yourself so you can provide this care safely and correctly at home. Remember that reading this book is not a substitute for medical training. Consult your doctor to find out what types of care to provide and which procedures to perform.

Personal Care

Hygiene is the term describing practices that we follow to keep our bodies clean and healthy. Grooming refers to such practices as caring for fingernails and hair. Hygiene and grooming activities, along with dressing, preparing meals, and eating, are activities of daily living (ADLs).

Some people who are ill may not have enough energy to care for themselves. Your may need to provide all personal care for your loved one. This personal care will include bathing, perineal care (care of the perineum, or area around, between, and including the genitals and anus), mouth care, hair care, nail care, shaving, dressing, and changing bed linens.

Your loved one may never again be able to care for himself, or he may regain strength and resume some or all of his personal care. Help him to be as independent as possible. This means helping him learn to care for himself and encouraging him to get back to his self-care routines as soon as he is able. Promoting independence is essential to caregiving.

We all have routines for personal care and activities of daily living and preferences for how these activities are done. These routines and preferences are important to us even when we are elderly, sick, or disabled. If you are unaware of your loved one's routines and preferences, ask her, and try to accommodate her choices (Fig. 9-1).

Before you begin any procedure or task, talk with your loved one about exactly what you will be doing. Ask if she would like to use the bathroom or bedpan first. Provide her with privacy. Let her make as many decisions as possible about when, where, and how a procedure is done. If she becomes tired, stop and take a short rest. After completing a procedure, ask if she would like anything else.

Personal care procedures give you an opportunity to observe the condition of her skin, mobility, flexibility, comfort level, mental state, and ability to perform ADLs. As you bathe her, for example, observe her skin for color, texture, temperature, and level of moisture. Is it pale, yellow, ashen, or

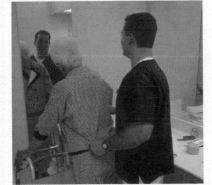

Fig. 9-1. Honoring your loved one's routines and preferences is an important part of promoting independence.

flushed? Are there blotches or a rash? Is the skin dry and flaky?

Is there any redness around bony areas? This is especially important to observe, as it could be a sign of a developing pressure sore. Pressure sores occur when the skin deteriorates from pressure and shearing. Eventually blood does not circulate properly and sores or ulcers form, swell, and may become infected.

Pressure sores usually occur on bony prominences, which are areas of the body where bone is close to the skin (Fig. 9-2). The skin here is at a much higher risk for skin breakdown.

Pressure sores are very painful and difficult to heal, and can lead to life-threatening infections. Prevention is very important. Use your personal care procedures as an opportunity to observe for and guard against pressure sores.

Many people will talk about any signs and symptoms they are experiencing while their personal care is administered. Your loved one may tell you that she has been itching or her skin feels dry. She may complain of numbness and tingling in a certain area of the body. Keep a small note pad nearby to record exactly how she describes these symptoms, or make your notes right after

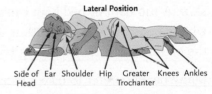

Lateral Position

Side of Head, Ear, Shoulder, Hip, Greater Trochanter, Knees, Ankles

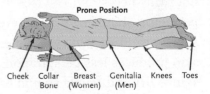

Prone Position

Cheek, Collar Bone, Breast (Women), Genitalia (Men), Knees, Toes

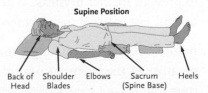

Supine Position

Back of Head, Shoulder Blades, Elbows, Sacrum (Spine Base), Heels

Fig. 9-2. Pressure sore danger zones.

the procedure. Report these comments to your doctor as appropriate.

You can also learn about her mental and emotional state at this time. Is she depressed or confused? Can she concentrate on an activity or hold a conversation?

Observe her overall physical health. Is she short of breath when moving or performing care? Does she tremble or shake? Is she having trouble using certain muscles or joints? Observe changes from her normal state. Is there a change in behavior, level of activity, skin color, movement, or anything else?

Bathing

Bathing promotes good health and well-being by removing perspiration, dirt, oil, and dead skin cells that accumulate on the skin. A tub bath or bed bath can also be relaxing. For someone who is bed-bound, a bed bath is an excellent time for moving the extremities and increasing body movement and circulation.

Many people prefer to take a bath or shower daily, but this is not really necessary. The face, hands, axillae (underarms), and perineum should be washed every day. A complete bath or shower can be taken every other day or even less often. Older skin produces less perspiration and oil. Elderly people whose skin is dry and fragile should bathe only once or twice a week to prevent further dryness. When bathing an older person, be careful not to wash the skin too vigorously.

Before bathing or assisting with bathing, make sure the temperature of the room is comfortably warm. Remove any loose rugs that do not have slip-resistant rubber backings. Familiarize yourself with available safety and assistive devices. Never leave an elderly person alone in the bathtub. Never use bath oils; they make the tub slippery and can cause falls.

Gloves may be worn when assisting with bathing. Or you may choose to wear gloves only for perineal care or if broken skin is present. As always, follow the doctor's instructions.

Using assistive devices in bathing

Assistive devices, such as a transfer belt or lift, tub chair, and safety bars, make bathing easier and safer for both your loved one and you. An occupational therapist (OT) can teach you transfer techniques for getting a person safely into and out of the bathtub. The job of the occupational therapist is to help clients improve their abilities to perform ADLs.

Transfer belts attach around the waist for safety during transfers or assisting with walking (ambulation). The belt can make it easier to help someone into and out of the tub. Mechanical lifts are another way to transfer a person from bed to a wheelchair or tub chair and back. More information about transfer belts and mechanical lifts is found in chapter 10.

A tub chair, shower chair, or bath bench is a sturdy chair or bench designed to be placed in a bathtub (Fig. 9-3). It is water- and slip-resistant. The chair or bench enables someone who cannot get

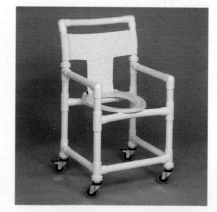

Fig. 9-3. One type of shower chair. (Photo courtesy of Innovative Products Unlimited)

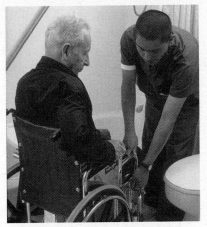

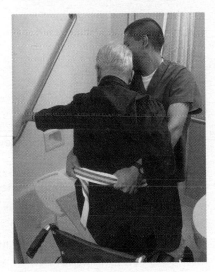

down into a tub or is too weak to stand in a shower to bathe in the tub rather than in bed. Safety bars, or grab bars, are installed in and near the tub and near the toilet to provide something to hold onto while changing position.

Helping a person transfer to the bathtub

As was mentioned in chapter 5, you will need to wear gloves for all procedures if you have broken skin on your hands or if there is broken skin on any area of the person's body that you will be touching. In the procedures in this chapter and all procedures that follow, gloves are only mentioned if they are always used in that procedure.

You may have to adapt this procedure to accommodate your loved one's level of strength.

Equipment: chair, transfer belt, if appropriate, shirt or robe to wear under transfer belt, slide board, if appropriate, tub chair, bath supplies (as listed in next procedure), gloves

1 Wash your hands.

2 Discuss what you will do.

3 Provide privacy.

4 Help your loved one to the bathroom. See chapter 10 for instructions for assisting with ambulation or transfers.

5 Seat him in a chair facing the bathtub and centered between the grab bars. If using a wheelchair, lock the brakes and raise the footrests (Fig. 9-4).

6 Ask him to place one leg at a time over the sides of the tub.

7 Have him hold onto the grab bars or the edge of the tub to bring himself to a sitting position on the edge of the tub. A slide board may be used to help him move from the chair to the tub. See chapter 10 for information on how to use a slide board to assist in transfers.

Fig. 9-4. Lock the brakes on a wheelchair before transferring a person to the bathtub.

8 Help him lower himself into the tub or onto the tub chair while holding onto the edge of the tub or grab bars. If necessary, hold him around the waist or have him wear a transfer belt (Fig. 9-5). If using a transfer belt to get in and out of the tub, he will need to wear a shirt or robe so the belt is not placed directly against his skin.

9 Reverse this procedure to help your loved one out of the tub. If he has trouble getting out of the tub, help him to his hands and knees. From that position, he can use the grab bar or the edge of the tub to pull himself up. You can also help by putting the transfer belt back on (over a robe).

Fig. 9-5.

If your loved one can get out of bed on her own to take a shower or bath, she will need a different level of assistance and supervision. Remember to allow as much independence and privacy as possible.

Helping a person who can walk to take a shower or tub bath

Equipment: two bath towels, washcloth, soap or other cleanser, bath thermometer (if available), rubber bath mat, tub or shower chair (if appropriate), table for bath supplies and bell (if she can bathe without assistance), non-skid bath rug, deodorant, powder, lotion and other toiletries, clean clothes or a robe, shoes or non-skid slippers, gloves

1 Wash your hands.

2 Discuss what you will do.

3 Provide privacy.

4 Clean tub or shower if necessary.

5 Place rubber mat on tub or shower floor. Set up tub or shower chair. Place skid-resistant bath rug on the floor next to the tub or shower.

6 Fill the tub with warm water (105° F to 110° F on the bath thermometer, or test the water on the inside of your wrist for comfort) or adjust the shower water temperature. Have your loved one test the water temperature to make sure it is comfortable for her.

7 Ask her to undress; assist as needed. Help her transfer to the bathtub or step in the shower. If you can leave her to bathe alone, place the bathing supplies on a small table within her reach (Fig. 9-6). Place a bell or other signal on the table and tell her to signal when you are needed. Tell her not to add more hot or warm water and not to remain in the tub for more than twenty minutes. Do not lock the bathroom door. Check on her every five minutes. If

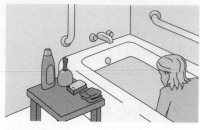

Fig. 9-6.

she is weak, stay with her in the bathroom. Otherwise, you can remake her bed while she is in the tub.

8 For a shower, stay with her and assist with washing hard-to-reach areas. Watch for signs of fatigue.

9 If she needs more assistance in the bath or shower, help her wash herself. Always move from clean areas to dirty areas to avoid spreading dirt into areas that have already been washed. Make sure all soap is rinsed off so the skin does not become dry or irritated.

10 Assist with shampooing hair, if necessary (see Procedure 4). Make sure all shampoo is rinsed out of hair.

11 When the bath or shower is finished, help her get out of the tub or shower. Wrap her in a towel. Have her sit in a chair or on the toilet seat and provide her with another towel for drying herself. Offer assistance in drying hard-to-reach places (Fig. 9-7). She may need help applying powder, deodorant, or lotion. If necessary, help her get dressed.

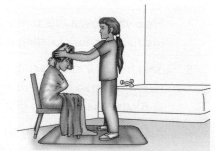

Fig. 9-7.

12 If she is tired after the bath or shower, help her back to the bed. Other personal care, such as mouth care, can be done later or while she is in bed.

13 Clean the tub and place soiled laundry (towels, washcloths, dirty clothes) in the laundry hamper.

14 Wash your hands.

15 Put away supplies.

16 Note any observations. Did you see any redness or whiteness on the skin? Was there any broken skin? How did your loved one tolerate bathing or showering? Has there been a change in abilities since the last bath or shower?

If your loved one cannot get out of bed, you will need to help him to take a bath in bed. Remember that independence and privacy are still important; let him do as much as he can for himself and never expose more of his body than is necessary.

Assisting with a bed bath

Equipment: basin, bath thermometer (if available), soap, two washcloths, two or three towels, orangewood stick or nail brush (if available), lotion, powder, deodorant, soft cotton blanket or a large towel, clean clothes, clean bed linens, gloves (two pairs)

1 Wash your hands.

2 Discuss what you will do.

3 Provide privacy.

4 If bed is adjustable, adjust it to a safe working level, usually waist high. If bed is movable, lock bed wheels.

5 Be sure the room is a comfortable temperature and there are no drafts.

6 Ask your loved one to remove glasses and jewelry and put them in a safe place. Offer to bring a bedpan or urinal for him to use before the bath (see Procedures 13 and 14 in this chapter).

7 Place a soft cotton blanket or towel over him (Fig. 9-8). Ask him to hold on to it as you remove the top sheet and blanket. Check the sheets for spills or body discharges.

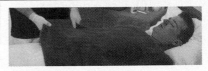

Fig. 9-8.

8 Fill the basin with warm water. Check the temperature with a bath thermometer or against the inside of your wrist. Water temperature should be between 105° F and 110° F on a thermometer. Allow him to feel the temperature to see if it is comfortable for him. During the bath, change the water when it becomes too cool, soapy, or dirty.

9 Ask your loved one to move to the side of the bed near where you are standing; assist if necessary. Ask and assist him to participate in washing. Uncover only one part of the body at a time. Place a towel under the body part being washed. Wash, rinse, and dry one part of the body at a time, starting at the head and working down. Complete the front first.

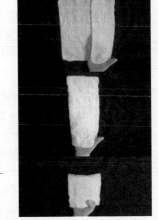

10 Fold the washcloth over your hand like a mitt and hold it in place with your thumb (Fig. 9-9).

Fig. 9-9.

11 Before you put soap on the cloth, wash your loved one's eyes and face. Start with the eye farther away from you;

wipe from the inner corner, near the bridge of the nose, to the outer corner (Fig. 9-10). Use a different section of the washcloth for the other eye. Wash the face from the

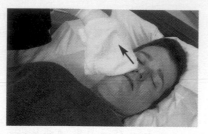

Fig. 9-10.

middle outward using firm but gentle strokes. Wash the neck and ears and behind the ears. Rinse and pat dry. If his face is oily, ask if you may use soap. Some people prefer creams for cleansing their face.

12   Remove his top clothing and cover him with the cotton bath blanket and towel again. Expose one arm. Using long strokes from the shoulder down to the elbow, wash the upper arm and underarm with a soapy washcloth. Rinse and pat dry. After washing the elbow, wash, rinse, and dry from the elbow down to the wrist (Fig. 9-11).

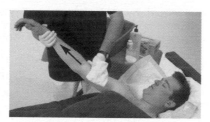

Fig. 9-11.

13   To wash the hand, place it in the basin. Wash the hand and clean under the nails with an orangewood stick or nail brush, if available (Fig. 9-12). Rinse and pat dry. Provide nail care (see Procedure 7) as needed. Do not provide nail care for a person who is diabetic. Repeat steps 12 and 13 for the other arm and hand. Put

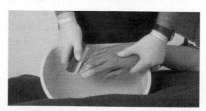

Fig. 9-12.

moisturizing lotion on the elbows and hands.

14   Place the towel once again across your loved one's chest and pull the blanket down to his waist. Lift the towel only enough to wash the chest, rinse it, and pat dry. Be sure to wash under a woman's breasts and check the skin in this area for signs of irritation and chafing. Ask if you may apply powder to the skin under the breasts after the area is dry.

15   Fold the cotton blanket down so that it still covers the pubic area. Wash and rinse the abdomen and pat dry. If your loved one has an ostomy, or opening in the abdomen for getting rid of body wastes, provide skin care around the opening. Chapter 7 includes more information about ostomies. Cover with the towel. Pull the cotton blanket up to his chin and remove the towel.

16   Expose one leg and place a towel under it. Wash the thigh, using long, downward strokes, then rinse and pat dry. Repeat this step from the knee to the ankle (Fig. 9-13).

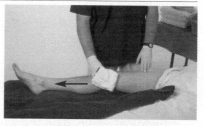

Fig. 9-13.

17   Place another towel under the foot and transfer the basin to the towel. Place his foot into the basin and wash the foot and between the toes (Fig. 9-14).

18   Perform nail care as needed (see Procedure 7), unless your loved one is diabetic. Rinse the foot

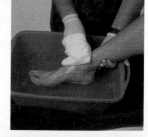

Fig. 9-14.

and pat dry, making sure the area between the toes is dry. Apply lotion to the foot, especially at the heels. Repeat steps 17 and 18 for the other leg and foot.

19 Help him move to the center of the bed and turn onto his side so his back is facing you. If the bed has rails, raise the rail on the opposite side for safety. Fold the cotton blanket away from his back. Place a towel lengthwise next to the back. Wash the back, neck, and buttocks with long, downward strokes (Fig. 9-15). Rinse and pat dry. Apply powder or lotion.

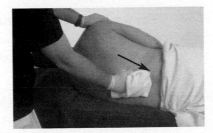

Fig. 9-15.

20 Place the towel under the buttocks and upper thighs. Help your loved one turn onto his back. If he is able to complete the bath by washing the perineal area himself, place a basin of clean, warm water within reach, along with a washcloth and towel. Leave the room for five minutes to provide privacy. If a urinary catheter is in place, remind him not to pull or disturb it.

21 If your loved one cannot provide perineal care, you must do it for him. Wearing gloves will prevent your hands from coming in contact with body secretions. Provide privacy at all times. Use clean water and a clean washcloth.

22 **For a woman**, always wash the perineum with soap and water from front to back, using single strokes (Fig. 9-16). Do not wash from the back to the front, as this may cause infection. First wipe the center of the perineum, then wipe each side. Use a clean area of the washcloth for each stroke. Spread the labia majora,

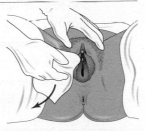

Fig. 9-16.

the outside folds of perineal skin that protect the urinary meatus and the vaginal opening. Wipe from front to back on each side. Wipe down the middle. Rinse the area in the same way. Ask her to turn on her side, then wash and rinse the anal area. Dry the perineum thoroughly and cover her with the cotton blanket.

For a man, if he is uncircumcised, retract the foreskin first. Hold the penis by the shaft and wash in a circular motion from the top down to the base (Fig. 9-17). Rinse the penis, then rinse the washcloth and wash the scrotum and groin. The groin is the area from the pubis to the upper thighs. Rinse and pat dry. Rinse the washcloth again. Ask him to turn on his side, then wash the anal area without contaminating the perineal area. Rinse and pat dry. Cover him with the cotton blanket.

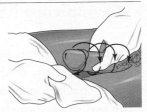

Fig. 9-17.

23 Place soiled washcloths and towels in the hamper or laundry basket. Dispose of the dirty bath water in the toilet. Discard your gloves into a trash receptacle. If time permits, a bed bath is a good time to give a back rub (Procedure 5).

24 Provide deodorant. Place a towel over the pillow and brush or comb hair (Procedure 6 in this chapter). Help your loved one put on clean clothing and get into a comfortable position with good body alignment.

25 If he uses a signaling device, place it within reach. Remove the bath supplies and wash and store everything. Change the bed sheets and blanket. Place used bed linens in the hamper or laundry basket.

26 Wash your hands.

27 Note any observations. Did you notice any redness or whiteness on the skin? Was there any broken skin? How was the bath or shower tolerated? Did he describe any symptoms? Has there been a change in his abilities since the last bath or shower?

Shampooing hair

A person who can get out of bed may have his hair shampooed in the sink, tub, or shower. For a person who cannot get out of bed, special rubber or plastic troughs exist for washing the hair in bed. These troughs fit under the head and neck and have a spout or hose that drains the water into a basin at the side of the bed; they should be available at a home medical supply store. You may also use a plastic garbage bag formed around a rolled towel.

Equipment: shampoo, hair conditioner, washcloth, pitcher, plastic cup or hand-held shower or sink attachment, gloves, chair (for washing hair in sink), large garbage bag or plastic sheet (for washing hair in sink), towel (two towels if washing hair in bed), cotton blanket (for washing hair in bed), waterproof mat (for washing hair in bed), trough or garbage bag and extra towel (for washing hair in bed), catch basin (for washing hair in bed)

1 Wash your hands.

2 Discuss what you will do.

3 Provide privacy.

4 If bed is adjustable, adjust it to a safe working level, usually waist high. If bed is movable, lock bed wheels.

5 Position your loved one and wet his hair.

a. **For washing hair in the sink**, seat him in a chair covered with plastic. Place a pillow under the plastic to support his head and neck. Have him lean his head back toward the sink. Give him a folded washcloth to hold over his forehead or eyes. Wet his hair using a plastic cup or a hand-held sink attachment.

b. **For washing hair in the tub**, have him tilt his head back. Give him a folded washcloth to hold over his forehead or eyes. Wet hair using a plastic cup or hand-held shower attachment.

c. **For washing hair in the shower**, have him turn so his back is toward the showerhead. Ask him to tilt his head back. Direct the flow of water over the hair to wet it.

d. **For washing hair in bed**, arrange the supplies within reach on a nearby table.

6 Remove all pillows, and place him in a flat position. Place a waterproof sheet or mat beneath his head and shoulders. Cover him with the cotton blanket, and fold back the top sheet and regular blankets. Place the trough under his head, then connect the trough to the catch basin. Using the pitcher, pour enough water on the hair to make it thoroughly wet.

7 Apply a small amount of shampoo to your hands and rub them together. Using both hands, massage the shampoo to a lather in the hair. With your fingertips, massage the scalp in a circular motion from front to back (Fig. 9-18).

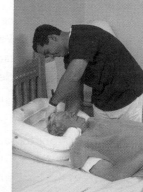

Fig. 9-18.

8 Rinse the hair in the same way you wet it. Repeat the shampoo and rinse. Use conditioner if desired. Be sure to

rinse the hair thoroughly to prevent the scalp from getting dry and itchy.

9   Wrap your loved one's hair in a towel. If shampooing at the sink, return him to an upright position. If shampooing in the bath or shower, assist him from the tub or shower as in earlier procedure. If shampooing in bed, remove the trough. Using the washcloth or a face towel, dry his head and neck.

10   Remove the hair towel and comb or brush hair (see procedure later in the chapter).

11   Dry the hair with a hair dryer on the low setting. Style the hair as he prefers.

12   Wash and store equipment. Put soiled towels and washcloth in the hamper or laundry basket.

13   Wash your hands.

14   Note your observations. How did your loved one tolerate having his hair washed? Was he able to help? Have his abilities changed since the last time his hair was washed?

Back rubs are often given after baths. A back rub can help a person to relax. It can make him more comfortable and increase circulation (Fig. 9-19). It also provides a good opportunity for you to observe your loved one's skin. Examples of things to watch for while giving a back rub include discolored areas and broken skin.

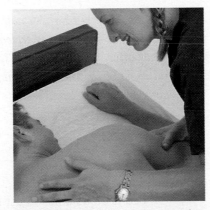

Fig. 9-19. Back rubs increase circulation and can help a person relax.

Giving a back rub

Equipment: body lotion, towel, cotton blanket

1   Wash your hands.

2   Discuss what you will do.

3   Provide privacy.

4   If bed is adjustable, adjust it to a safe working level, usually waist high. If bed is movable, lock bed wheels.

5   Have your loved one lie on his stomach; if this is uncomfortable, have him lie on his side. Cover him with a cotton blanket and fold back the bed covers. Expose his back to the middle of the buttocks. If he is positioned on his side, place the towel on the bed along the length of his back. Back rubs can also be given with a person sitting up.

6   Pour the lotion on your hands and rub them together to spread it. You may want to warm the lotion and your hands first. Immerse the lotion in warm water for five minutes and run your hands under warm water. Mention that the lotion may still feel cool. Always put the lotion on your hands rather than directly on the skin.

7   Place your hands on each side of the upper part of the buttocks. Make long, smooth upward strokes with both hands along each side of the spine, up to the shoulders (Fig. 9-20). Circle your hands outward and then move back along the outer

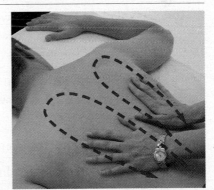

Fig. 9-20.

edges of the back. At the buttocks, make another circle and move your hands back up to the shoulders. Without taking your hands from his skin, repeat this motion for three to five minutes.

8   Next, make kneading motions with the first two fingers and thumb of each hand. Place them at the base of the spine and move upward simultaneously along each side of the spine, applying downward pressure. Follow the same direction as with the long smooth strokes, circling at shoulders and buttocks (Fig. 9-21).

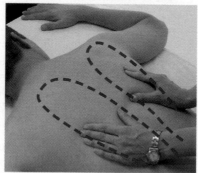

Fig. 9-21.

9   Gently massage bony areas (spine, shoulder blades, hip-bones) with circular motions of your fingertips. Gentle massage stimulates circulation and helps prevent skin damage. If any of these areas are red, massage around them rather than on them. The redness indicates that the skin is irritated and fragile.

10   Let your loved one know when you are almost done. Finish with long, smooth strokes like the ones you used at the beginning of the massage.

11   Dry the back if extra lotion remains on it. If desired, apply powder to the back to allow better movement against the sheets.

12   Remove the cotton blanket and towel.

13   Help your loved one get dressed.

14   Help him into a comfortable position.

15   Store the lotion and put dirty linens in the hamper.

16   Wash your hands.

17   Note observations. Did he appear comfortable during the back rub? Did you observe any reddened areas, whiteness, or broken skin?

Grooming

Your loved one has probably been taking care of her own grooming tasks for most of her life. She has certain ways that she prefers these tasks to be done. She may be embarrassed or depressed because she now needs help with these tasks that she has done for herself for so long. Remember to always allow her to do all that she can for herself. Your gentleness and respect will help her to maintain her dignity and feel good about herself.

Combing or brushing hair

Equipment: *comb, brush, or hair pick, bath towel, mirror, hair lotion or oil if desired, detangler, leave-in conditioner, or rubbing alcohol and cotton ball if the hair is tangled, accessories such as barrettes, bobby pins, small combs, or coated rubber bands, depending on style preference*

1   Wash your hands.

2   Discuss what you will do.

3   Provide privacy.

4   If bed is adjustable, adjust it to a safe working level, usually waist high. If bed is movable, lock bed wheels.

5   If she is confined to bed, raise the head of the bed and use a backrest or pillows to raise her head and shoulders. Place the towel under her head. If she is ambulatory, provide a comfortable chair. Place the towel around her shoulders.

6   Brush two-inch sections of hair at a time. Brush from roots to ends (Fig. 9-22).

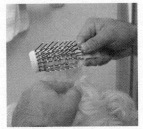

Fig. 9-22.

7   If the hair is tangled, work on the tangles first. Put a small amount of detangler or leave-in conditioner or a small amount of alcohol on the tangles. Hold the lock of hair just above the tangle so you don't pull at the scalp, and gently comb or brush through the tangle.

8   A person who has dry, brittle hair may require a special treatment with oil or hair lotion. Those with hair that is tightly curled may use a comb with large teeth or a pick.

9   Style hair as your loved one prefers (Fig. 9-23).

10 Remove the towel and shake excess hair in the wastebasket. Place the soiled towel in the hamper. Store supplies. Remove your gloves.

11 Wash your hands.

12 Note any observations.

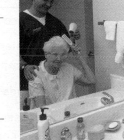

Fig. 9-23.

Providing fingernail care

Equipment: *orangewood stick, emery board, small basin or bowl, washcloth, lotion, cuticle softener or remover, bath towel, soap (if*

she uses nail polish, you will need nail polish, nail polish remover, cotton balls)

1   Wash your hands.

2   Discuss what you will do.

3   Provide privacy.

4   If bed is adjustable, adjust it to a safe working level, usually waist high. If bed is movable, lock bed wheels.

5   If necessary, remove nail polish with a cotton ball soaked with nail polish remover.

6   Fill the basin halfway with warm water. Test water temperature with your wrist to ensure that it is safe and comfortable. Have your loved one check the water temperature.

7   Soak her fingernails in the water. If you need to soften the cuticles to push them back, add a cuticle softener to the water or apply it to the cuticles. Soak all fingertips for two to four minutes.

8   Remove hands from water and wash them with a soapy washcloth. Rinse and dry them with a towel, making sure to dry between the fingers.

9   Place her hands on the towel. Gently push back the cuticles using the flat end of the orangewood stick or a towel.

10 Use the pointed end of the orangewood stick or a nail brush to remove dirt from under the nails (Fig. 9-24). Wipe the orangewood stick on the towel after cleaning under each nail. Wash her hands again and dry them thoroughly.

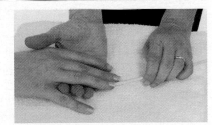

Fig. 9-24.

11   Shape fingernails with the emery board and apply lotion.

12   Discard the water and clean the basin. Place the towels in the laundry hamper and store supplies. If you raised an adjustable bed, return it to its lowest position.

13   Wash your hands.

14   Note any observations. Was there any redness, whiteness, or broken or discolored skin? Were there any differences in temperature of the hands or fingers?

If your loved one is diabetic, careful foot care is important. Because poor circulation occurs in diabetics, even a small cut on the foot could grow into a large wound, possibly even resulting in amputation. You should never clip the toenails of a person who is diabetic; a doctor or nurse must do it. There is more detailed information about diabetes in chapter 7.

Providing foot care

Equipment: *basin, pumice stone, two bath towels, washcloth, lotion, soap, clean socks, bath thermometer*

1   Wash your hands.

2   Discuss what you will do.

3   Provide privacy.

4   If bed is adjustable, adjust it to a safe working level, usually waist high. If bed is movable, lock bed wheels.

5   Fill the basin halfway with warm water. Test water temperature with the bath thermometer or with your wrist to ensure it is safe. Water temperature should be 105° F. Have your loved one check the water temperature. Adjust if nec-

essary. Place basin on a bath towel on the floor or at the foot of the bed.

6   Soak his feet for ten minutes. Add warm water to the basin if necessary.

7   Remove one foot from the basin. Smooth any rough areas with the pumice stone or a washcloth. Wash entire foot, including between the toes and around the nail beds, with a soapy washcloth.

8   Rinse entire foot, including between the toes. Thoroughly dry entire foot, including between the toes. Apply lotion. Do not attempt any further care of the toenails.

9   Repeat steps 7 and 8 for the other foot.

10   While you are giving foot care, observe the feet for sores, irritated or reddened areas (especially on the heels), any discoloration or darkening of the foot, discoloration of the toes or toenails, swelling, infection, or differences in temperature. Even if another person provides foot care, you should still observe for these signs of problems or illness on a regular basis.

11   Assist your loved one to replace his socks.

12   Discard the water and clean the basin. Put the towels in the laundry hamper and store supplies.

13   Wash your hands.

14   Record any observations. Was there any redness, whiteness, or broken or discolored skin? Were there any differences in temperature of the toes or feet?

Be sure your loved one wants you to shave him or help him shave before you begin. Put on gloves before helping someone shave, as the possibility of nicks means that your hands may come into contact with body fluids. There are several types of razor that can be used. A safety razor has a sharp blade with a special safety casing to help prevent cuts. It requires the use of shaving cream or soap. An electric razor is the safest and easiest to use and requires no soap or shaving cream. A disposable razor requires soap or shaving cream and is thrown away after use. Choose the one that he likes best or that best suits your needs.

Helping someone shave

Equipment: *clean safety razor, electric razor, or disposable razor, shaving cream or gel (if using a safety razor or disposable razor), basin filled with warm water (if using a safety razor or disposable razor), bath towel, washcloth, mirror, aftershave lotion, gloves*

1   Wash your hands.

2   Discuss what you will do.

3   Provide privacy.

4   If bed is adjustable, adjust it to a safe working level, usually waist high. If bed is movable, lock bed wheels.

5   Put on gloves.

6   Place the equipment on a table within your loved one's reach if he is shaving himself. If he is bedbound, use pillows or a backrest to help him sit up in a comfortable position. If he wears dentures, be sure they are in place. Place the towel across his chest.

7   If you are using an electric razor, use a small brush to clean it. Do not use an electric razor near any water source, when oxygen is in use, or for someone who has a pacemaker. Turn on the razor and shave the face, pulling the skin tight over the mouth and cheeks if necessary to

shave more smoothly. Shave the chin and under the chin (Fig. 9-25).

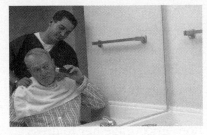

Fig. 9-25.

8   If you are using a safety razor, use a sharp blade. A dull blade is damaging to the skin. Soften the beard with a warm wet towel for a few minutes before shaving. Lather the face with shaving cream or gel and warm water. This makes shaving more comfortable. Shave in the direction of hair growth for a more comfortable and even shave. Use short strokes on the chin and longer strokes on the cheeks (Fig. 9-26). Rinse the blade frequently in the basin.

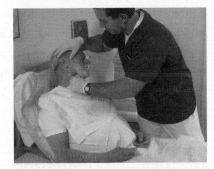

Fig. 9-26.

9   When you have finished, rinse the face with a warm, wet washcloth or let him use the washcloth himself. Offer him a mirror.

10   If he wants aftershave, moisten your palms with aftershave lotion and pat it onto his face.

11   Clean the equipment and store it. Dispose of the used disposable razor or blade. Put the towel and washcloth in the hamper or laundry basket. Remove and discard gloves.

12   Wash your hands.

13.   Note any observations.

Whenever possible, allow your loved one to choose her own clothing (Fig. 9-27). Check to ensure that it is clean, appropriate for the weather, and in good condition. Encourage her to dress in regular clothes during the day rather than in night-clothes. Wearing regular daytime clothing encourages more activity and less time in bed. Elastic-waist pants or skirts are easy to pull on over the legs and hips. Be sure the elastic waistband of underpants, slips, pantyhose, pants, or skirts fits comfortably at the waist. Clothing that is a size larger than normally worn is easier to put on. Consider these guidelines:

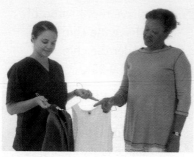

Fig. 9-27. Having your loved one choose her own clothing promotes independence and dignity.

GUIDELINES
Dressing and Undressing

Your loved one should do as much to dress or undress himself as possible. It may take longer, but it helps maintain independence and regain self-care skills. Ask where your assistance is needed.

Provide privacy. If he has just had a bath, cover him with a cotton bath blanket. Put on undergarments first. Never expose more of the body than necessary.

If there is weakness or paralysis on one side, place the weak arm or leg through the garment first, then the strong arm (Fig. 9-28). When undressing, do the opposite.

When putting on socks or stockings, roll or fold them down. They can then be slipped over the toes and foot and unrolled up into place on the leg. Make certain that toes, heels, and seams of socks or stockings are in the right place.

For a woman, make sure bra cups fit over the breasts. Front-fastening bras are easier for most women to manage by themselves. Bras that fasten in back can be put around the waist and fastened in front first, then turned around and pulled up, putting the arms through the straps last. This can be reversed for undressing.

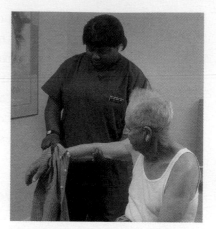

Fig. 9-28. When dressing, assist with the involved, or weaker, side first.

Several types of adaptive aids, such as long-handled hooks and pulls, are available to help maintain independence in dressing (Fig. 9-29). An occupational therapist can help you and your loved one learn to use these aids.

Oral Care

Oral care, care of the mouth, teeth, and gums, is per-

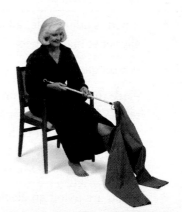

Fig. 9-29. One type of adaptive aid for dressing. (Photo courtesy of North Coast Medical, Inc., www.ncmedical.com, 800-821-9319)

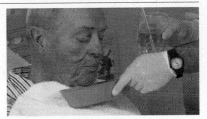

formed at least twice each day to cleanse the mouth of food particles and secretions. It should be done after breakfast and after the last meal or snack of the day. Oral care includes brushing the teeth and gums, flossing the teeth, and caring for dentures. When you perform or assist with oral care, take the opportunity to observe the mouth. Observe and report any of the following:

- irritation

- infection

- raised areas

- coated tongue

- ulcers, such as canker sores or small, painful, white sores

- flaky, white spots

- dry, cracked or chapped lips

- loose or decayed teeth

- swollen, bleeding, or whitish gums

- breath that smells bad or fruity

Assisting with oral care

Equipment: soft-bristled toothbrush, toothpaste or powder, glass of water, two towels, moisturizer for lips, basin and a drinking straw (if person is in bed), gloves

1 Wash your hands.

2 Discuss what you will do.

3 Provide privacy.

4 If bed is adjustable, adjust it to a safe working level, usually waist high. If bed is movable, lock bed wheels.

5 Put on gloves.

6 Remove any dental bridgework (Procedure 13 in this chapter explains how to remove dentures) or ask him to do so.

7 Put toothpaste on the toothbrush.

8 Gently brush the teeth, or help him do so. Use short strokes and brush back and forth on all surfaces. Gently brush the tongue as well.

9 Give him water to rinse the mouth and place the basin under his chin for him to spit it into (Fig. 9-30).

Fig. 9-30.

10 Replace any dental bridgework (Procedure 12 in this chapter explains how to reinsert dentures). Apply moisturizer to the lips.

11 Put the soiled towel in the laundry hamper. Pour the water from the basin into the toilet. Clean the basin and store supplies. Remove and discard your gloves.

12 Wash your hands.

13 Note any observations. Did you see any mouth ulcers or broken skin? What was the condition of the mucous membrane? Did the breath smell unusual?

Although an unconscious person is not eating, breathing through the mouth dries saliva in the mouth. Good mouth care needs to be performed more frequently to keep the mouth clean and moist. Swabs with a mixture of lemon juice and glycerine are traditionally used to soothe the gums but may further dry them if used too often. Mouthwash may be used in place of glycerine.

With an unconscious person, it is important to use as little liquid as possible when performing mouth care. Because the person's swallowing reflex is weak, he is at risk for aspiration. Aspiration is the inhalation of food or drink into the lungs, and it can cause pneumonia or death.

Always explain what you will do before beginning any procedure. A person who is unconscious may be able to hear you. Always speak as you would if he were conscious.

Performing oral care on an unconscious person

Equipment: cotton or sponge swabs, lemon glycerine swabs, padded tongue blade, mouthwash or a solution of hydrogen peroxide and water, basin, towel, glass of cool water, lip moisturizer, gloves

1	Wash your hands.
2	Discuss what you will do.
3	Provide privacy.
4	If bed is adjustable, adjust it to a safe working level, usually waist high. If bed is movable, lock bed wheels.
5	Put on gloves.
6	Turn your loved one's head to the side and place a towel under his cheek and chin. Place a small basin next to the cheek and chin to catch excess fluid.
7	Dip the plain cotton or sponge swab in the mouthwash. Do not dip a lemon glycerine swab in mouthwash.

8	Separate the upper and lower teeth with the padded tongue blade (Fig. 9-31). Using the swab, cleanse all surfaces in the mouth cavity, including the teeth and underneath the tongue. Remove debris with the swab. Repeat this step until the mouth is clean (Fig. 9-32).
9	Swab again with the lemon glycerine swab.
10	Remove the towel and basin. Pat lips or face dry if needed and apply lip moisturizer.
11	Place the towel in the laundry hamper. Clean the basin and store supplies. Remove and discard your gloves.
12	Wash your hands.
13	Note any observations. Did you see any mouth ulcers or other broken skin? What was the condition of the mucous membrane? Did the breath smell unusual?

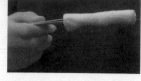

Fig. 9-31. To make a padded tongue blade, place two wooden tongue blades together and wrap the upper portion with gauze. Tape the gauze in place.

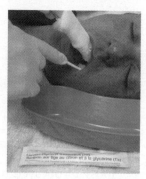

Fig. 9-32.

Flossing removes plaque and tartar buildup around the gum line and between the teeth. Teeth may be flossed immediately before or after they are brushed.

Flossing teeth

Equipment: about 18 inches of dental floss, glass of water, basin, face towel, gloves

1   Wash your hands.

2   Discuss what you will do.

3   Provide privacy.

4   If bed is adjustable, adjust it to a safe working level, usually waist high. If bed is movable, lock bed wheels.

5   Put on gloves.

6   Wrap the ends of the floss securely around your index fingers (Fig. 9-33).

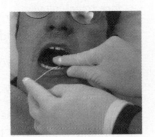

Fig. 9-33.

7   Starting with the back teeth, place the floss between teeth and move it down the surface of the tooth. Use a gentle sawing motion (Fig. 9-34). Continue to the gum line. At the gum line, curve the floss into a letter C, slip it gently into the space between the gum and tooth, and go back up, scraping the side of the tooth. Repeat this on the side of the other tooth (Fig. 9-35).

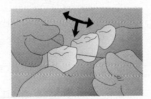

Fig. 9-34.

8   After every two or three teeth, unwind the floss from your fingers and move it so you are using a clean area. Floss all teeth.

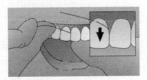

Fig. 9-35.

9   Occasionally offer water so that your loved one can rinse debris from the mouth into the basin.

10   When done flossing all teeth, offer a clean face towel.

11   Discard floss. Pour the water from the basin into the toilet and clean and store the basin. Put the soiled face towel in the laundry hamper. Remove and discard your gloves.

12   Wash your hands.

13   Note any observations.

If your loved one wears dentures, remember to ask how you can assist with denture care. Each person has her own preferences about when and how denture care should be done. Dentures are also very expensive; handle them carefully to avoid breaking or chipping them.

Assisting with denture care

Equipment: *denture cup for storage, denture cleaner or toothpaste, denture brush or soft toothbrush, two face towels, basin or sink, gauze squares, mouthwash or a cotton or sponge swab, gloves*

1   Wash your hands.

2   Discuss what you will do.

3   Provide privacy.

4   Put on gloves.

5   Line the sink or a basin with a face towel and fill with water. This will prevent the dentures from breaking if they fall into the sink.

6   Ask your loved one to remove her dentures and place them in the denture cup. If she is unable to remove them, do it yourself. Remove the lower denture first. The lower denture is easier to remove because it floats on the gum line of the lower jaw. Grasp the lower denture with a gauze square (for a good grip) and remove it. Place it in a denture cup filled with water.

Providing Personal Care

9

7   The upper denture is sealed by suction. Firmly grasp it with a gauze square and give a slight downward pull to break the suction. Turn it at an angle to take it out of the mouth.

8   Take the denture cup to the sink or basin. Apply denture cleanser to a denture brush or soft toothbrush, and brush the dentures under warm, running tap water to remove all material (Fig. 9-36). Do not use hot water or dentures may warp. Rinse out the denture cup and place the dentures in it.

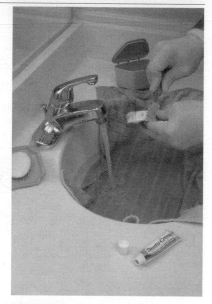

Fig. 9-36.

9   Some people prefer to clean their dentures with a soaking solution. Read the directions on the bottle to prepare the solution. Soak the dentures for the amount of time specified. Rinse and place them in the denture cup.

10 Store dentures in water or solution to prevent warping. To avoid accidentally discarding them, always store them in a labeled denture cup when not being worn.

11 Offer mouthwash or a swab to cleanse the mouth.

12 Clean and store equipment. Remove your gloves.

13 Wash your hands.

14 Note any observations.

Ask your loved one if she needs your assistance in inserting dentures. Remember to be very careful to avoid dropping or damaging them.

Reinserting dentures

Equipment: *denture cup with dentures, denture cream or adhesive, face towel, gloves*

1   Wash your hands.

2   Discuss what you will do.

3   Provide privacy.

4   If bed is adjustable, adjust it to a safe working level, usually waist high. If bed is movable, lock bed wheels.

5   Put on gloves.

6   Position your loved one as for brushing teeth; help her into as upright a position as possible.

7   Apply denture cream or adhesive to the dentures if needed.

8   Ask her to open mouth. Insert the upper denture into the mouth by turning it at an angle. Straighten it and press it firmly and evenly onto the upper gum line (Fig. 9-37).

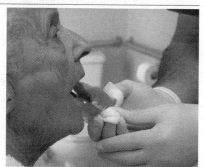

Fig. 9-37.

9   Insert the lower denture onto the gum line of the lower jaw and press firmly.

10 Offer a face towel.

11 Rinse and store the denture cup. Remove and discard gloves.

12 Wash your hands.

13 Note any observations.

Hearing Aids

There are many different types of hearing aids (Fig. 9-38). Follow the manufacturer's directions for cleaning a hearing aid. In general, use a little soap and water on a cloth, cotton swab, or pipe cleaner to keep the earpiece free of wax and dirt. Do not submerge the hearing aid or allow the section that houses the battery to get wet. Handle the hearing aid carefully. Do not drop it. Keep the hearing aid in a safe place when it is not being worn. Keep an extra battery on hand.

Toileting

A person who is unable to get out of bed to go to the bathroom may use a bedpan or a urinal. A fracture pan, which is flatter than a regular bedpan, is used for someone who cannot raise his hips onto a regular bedpan (Fig. 9-39). Women will use a bedpan for urination and bowel movements; men will generally use a urinal for urination and a bedpan for bowel movements (Fig. 9-40).

If your loved one is able to get out of bed, he may still need help walking to the bathroom and using the toilet. You may wish to provide

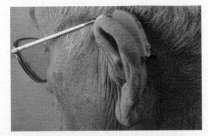

Fig. 9-38. One type of hearing aid.

a portable commode, a chair with a toilet seat and a removable container underneath. In homes where the bathroom is on a different floor, portable commodes are very useful. If your loved one needs assistance to get to the bathroom or use the toilet or commode, offer help frequently. This can prevent accidents and embarrassment. Toilets can be fitted with raised seats to make it easier for a person with limited mobility to get up and down. Handrails can also be installed next to the toilet.

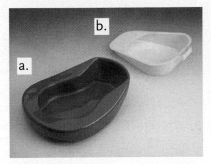

Fig. 9-39. a) Standard pan and b) fracture pan.

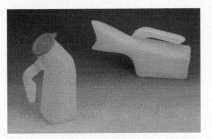

Fig. 9-40. Two types of urinals.

Assisting in using a bedpan

Equipment: *bedpan, bedpan cover (newspaper or washable cloth), protective plastic or latex sheet, talcum powder or cornstarch, cotton bath blanket, toilet paper, disposable or regular washcloths, gloves*

1 Wash your hands.

2 Discuss what you will do.

3 Provide privacy.

4 If bed is adjustable, adjust it to a safe working level, usually waist high. If bed is movable, lock bed wheels.

5 Put on gloves.

6   Warm the outside of the bedpan with warm water in the bathroom. Cover it when you bring it to the bed. Dust the top of the bedpan with talcum powder to prevent it from sticking to the skin. Do not use talcum powder if there are open sores on the buttocks or genitals. If a stool or urine sample is not needed, place a few sheets of toilet paper in the bedpan to make cleanup easier.

7   Cover your loved one with the cotton bath blanket. Ask him to hold it while you pull down the top covers underneath it.

8   Place a protective sheet under him. To do this, have him roll toward you. If he is unable to do this unassisted, you must roll him (see chapter 10). Be sure he cannot roll off the bed. Move to the empty side of the bed and place the protective sheet on the area where he will lie on his back. The side of the protective sheet nearest him should be fanfolded (folded several times into pleats) (Fig. 9-41). Ask him to roll onto his back, or roll him as you did before. Unfold the rest of the sheet so it completely covers the area under and around his hips (Fig. 9-42).

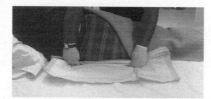

Fig. 9-41.

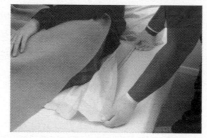

Fig. 9-42.

9   Ask him to remove his undergarments or help him do so.

10   While he is lying on his back, adjust the bed or use pillows to prop up the upper body. Place the bedpan near his hips with the open end facing the foot of the bed.

11   Slide the bedpan under his hips. Ask him to help by raising your loved one's hips at the count of three (Fig. 9-43). If he cannot do this himself, place your arm under the small of his back and tell him to push with his heels and hands on your signal as you raise his hips (Fig. 9-44). If he cannot help you in any way, keep the bed flat and roll him onto the far side. Slip the bedpan under the hips and roll him back onto the bedpan. Then prop him into a semi-sitting position using pillows.

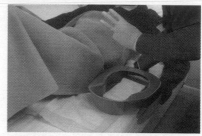

Fig. 9-43.

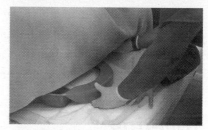

Fig. 9-44.

12   Check the bedpan to be certain it is in the correct position. Make sure the bath blanket is still covering your loved one. Provide him with toilet paper, disposable washcloths, and a bell or other way to call you. Tell him you will return when called. Make sure he is comfortable before you leave.

13   If he is unable to clean his anal area and the rest of the perineum, you must do this. With gloves on, help him roll onto his side. Use the toilet paper to clean the perineal area first. For a woman, wipe from front to back. Use one disposable washcloth to cleanse the front part of the perineum and another to cleanse the anal area.

14   Wrap the toilet paper and disposable washcloths in a plas-

tic bag and discard them. Dry the perineal area with a towel and place the towel in a hamper. Remove and discard your gloves. Immediately replace them with a clean pair.

15 Offer a wet washcloth and soap and water for washing your loved one's hands. Cover him and remove the cotton bath blanket. Help him put on undergarments.

16 Cover the bedpan and take it to the bathroom. Empty it carefully into the toilet and flush. If you notice anything unusual about the stool or urine (such as the presence of blood), do not discard it. Remove and discard your gloves, wash your hands, and notify the doctor. He or she may ask you to save a specimen (chapter 11 describes how to collect stool specimens). Put on new gloves.

17 Turn the faucet on with a paper towel. Rinse the bedpan with cold water and empty it into the toilet. Clean the bedpan with hot, soapy water and store it.

18 Remove and discard gloves.

19 Wash your hands.

20 Note the time of the elimination, the contents, and any observations.

Your loved one may ask for the urinal, or you may ask if he needs it at regular times. Remember that your loved one may be embarrassed about needing help to use a urinal; provide him with as much privacy as you can.

Assisting in using a urinal

Equipment: *urinal, protective plastic or latex sheet, cotton bath blanket, soap, washcloth, basin, towel, gloves*

1 Wash your hands.

2 Discuss what you will do.

3 Provide privacy.

4 If bed is adjustable, adjust it to a safe working level, usually waist high. If bed is movable, lock bed wheels.

5 Put on gloves.

6 Place a protective pad under the buttocks and hips.

7 Hand your loved one the urinal. If he is not able to help himself, place the urinal between his legs and position the penis inside the urinal (Fig. 9-45). Replace covers.

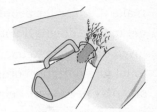

8 Give him a bell or another way to call you. Leave the room and close the door.

Fig. 9-45.

9 When he signals that he is finished, remove the urinal or have him hand it to you. Follow the correct procedure if a specimen has been ordered (see chapter 11). Discard urine in the toilet. Use a paper towel to turn on the faucet. Rinse the urinal with cold water and store it.

10 Remove and discard your gloves. Wash your hands.

11 Give your loved one a washcloth, soap, and water to wash his hands.

12 After taking the washcloth from him and placing it aside (to be washed separately from other laundry), wash your hands again.

13 Note the time, the amount of urine (if monitoring intake and output), and any other observations.

Some people who are able to get out of bed but cannot walk to the bathroom may use a portable commode. A portable commode is a chair with a toilet seat and a re-movable container under-neath (Fig. 9-46). Toilets can be fitted with raised seats to make it easier for people to get up and down. If your loved one needs to use the toilet or a portable commode,

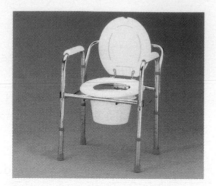

Fig. 9-46. A portable commode can be used for people who can get out of bed but may not be able to move to the bathroom easily. (Photo courtesy of Nova Ortho Med, Inc.)

she may need your help. She may ask for the portable com-mode, or you may need to offer it frequently.

Assisting with use of the toilet or a portable commode

Equipment: toilet paper, disposable washcloths, soap, washcloth, basin (if using portable commode), gloves

1   Wash your hands.

2   Discuss what you will do.

3   Provide privacy.

4   If bed is adjustable, adjust it to a safe working level, usu-ally waist high. If bed is movable, lock bed wheels.

5   Put on gloves.

6   Help your loved one out of bed and to the bathroom or portable commode.

7   If needed, help her remove clothing and sit on toilet seat.

8   Provide privacy and leave the room or area. Close the door, but do not lock it. Provide a bell or another way for her to call you.

9   Return when she calls you. If assistance is needed to clean the perineal area, provide it. Remember to wipe a woman's perineal area from front to back. Use disposable washcloths if necessary. Dispose of these in the toilet or in the wastebasket if they are not flushable. If your gloves be-come soiled, discard them and put on fresh gloves.

10   Help her up and be sure she washes her hands before re-turning to bed. Use the sink or a basin, soap, and a washcloth.

11   When using a portable commode, remove waste container and empty it into the toilet unless a specimen is needed or her urine is being measured for intake/output monitoring (see chapter 12). Clean the container as you would a bed-pan, rinsing first with cold water and then washing with hot water and cleanser.

12   Remove and discard your gloves.

13   Wash your hands.

14   Note any observations.

Good perineal care is essential to prevent infection, skin irrita-tion, and odor. A person who is incontinent needs regular and thorough perineal care. Never let embarrassment keep you from providing good perineal care. You can protect privacy and dignity without neglecting perineal care.

Always wear gloves when providing or assisting with perineal care. Specific instructions for perineal care are found earlier in this chapter in the procedure for assisting with a bed bath.

Wastes such as urine and feces can carry infection. Always dispose of wastes in the toilet; be careful not to spill or splash. Wear gloves when handling bedpans, urinals, or basins that contain wastes, including dirty bath water. Wash these containers thoroughly, and use a disinfectant. Then remove your gloves and wash your hands. Put on a new pair of gloves if you are not finished providing care.

Washcloths used to clean the perineal area must be washed in hot water. Handle such laundry carefully, with gloves. Wash it separately from other family laundry. Disposable washcloths may or may not be flushable; read the package to be sure. If they are not flushable, dispose of them in a waste container lined with a plastic bag. Remove and replace the plastic bag frequently to prevent odors.

Sleep and Bedmaking

Sleep and rest are important needs that must be met. Sleep provides us with new cells and energy. Many elderly persons have sleep and rest problems. Many things can affect sleeping patterns, such as fear, anxiety, noise, diet, medications, and illness. If your loved one complains of lack of sleep, observe for such things as:

- sleeping too much during the day

- too much caffeine late in the afternoon or evening

- dressing in night clothes during the day

- eating too late at night

- refusing medication prescribed for sleep

- medications with side effects that disturb sleep

- keeping the TV or light on late at night

- pain

If your loved one spends much or all of her time in bed, careful bedmaking is essential to comfort, cleanliness, and health. Linens should always be changed after personal care procedures such as bed baths. Also change them any time bedding or sheets are damp, soiled, or in need of straightening. It is important that bed linens be changed frequently for three reasons:

1. Sheets that are damp, wrinkled, or bunched up are uncomfortable. They may prevent rest or sleep.

2. Microorganisms thrive in moist, warm environments. Bedding that is damp or unclean may encourage infection and disease.

3. A person who spends long hours in bed is at risk for pressure sores. Sheets that do not lie flat under the body increase this risk by affecting the circulation.

GUIDELINES
Bedmaking

When collecting clean linen to make a bed, hold it away from your clothes. If linen touches your clothes, it may become contaminated.

Do not shake soiled linen. This may spread airborne contaminants.

Check linens for things like dentures, hearing aids, and glasses before removing them from the bed for laundering.

If your loved one cannot get out of bed, you must change the linens with him in bed. When making the bed, use a wide stance with your knees bent. Avoid bending from the waist, especially when tucking sheets or blankets under the mattress; mattresses can be heavy. Bend your knees to avoid injury. It is easier to make an unoccupied bed than one with someone in it. If your loved one can be moved to a chair or other comfortable spot, your job will be easier.

Making an occupied bed

Equipment: clean linen, mattress pad, fitted or flat bottom sheet, waterproof bed protector if needed, cotton draw sheet, flat top sheet, blanket(s), pillowcase(s), gloves (if you're going to be touching linens soiled with body fluids)

1   Wash your hands.

2   Discuss what you will do.

3   Provide privacy.

4   If bed is adjustable, adjust it to a safe working level, usually waist high. If bed is movable, lock bed wheels.

5   Put on gloves.

6   Place clean linen on clean surface within reach (e.g., bedside stand, overbed table, or chair).

7   Loosen top linen from the end of the bed or working side. Cover your loved one with a cotton bath blanket or the loosened top sheet on the bed.

8   Raise side rail, if there is one, on far side of bed. After raising side rail, help your loved one turn onto his side, moving away from you toward raised side rail (Fig. 9-47). If the bed has no side rail, use pillows, chair backs, or another

family member or helper to be sure your loved one does not fall from the bed while you are making it.

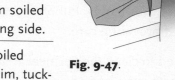

9   Loosen bottom soiled linen on working side.

10   Roll bottom soiled linen toward him, tucking it snugly against his back.

Fig. 9-47.

11   Place and tuck in clean bottom linen, finishing with bottom sheet free of wrinkles. If you are using a flat bottom sheet, leave enough overlap on each end to tuck under the mattress. If the sheet is only long enough to tuck in at one end, tuck it in securely at the top of the bed. Make hospital corners to keep the bottom sheet wrinkle-free (Fig. 9-48).

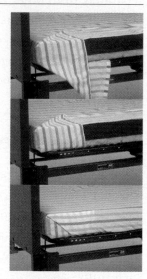

12   Smooth the bottom sheet out toward him. Be sure there are no wrinkles in the mattress pad. Roll the extra material toward him and tuck it under his body.

Fig. 9-48.

13   If using a waterproof pad, unfold and center it on the bed. Tuck the side near you under the mattress. Smooth it out toward him and tuck as you did with the sheet.

14   If using a draw sheet, place it on the bed. Tuck in on your side, smooth, and tuck as you did with the other bedding.

15 Assist your loved one to turn onto clean bottom sheet toward you. Protect him from any soiled matter on the old linens. Raise side rail nearest you, if there is one.

16 Move to the other side of the bed and lower the side rail, if applicable.

17 Loosen the soiled linen and roll it from the head to the foot of the bed, avoiding contact with your skin and clothes. Place it in a hamper or basket. Never put it on the floor or furniture; never shake it. Soiled bed linens are full of microorganisms that should not be spread to other parts of the room.

18 Pull and tuck in clean bottom linen just like the other side, finishing with bottom sheet free of wrinkles (Fig. 9-49).

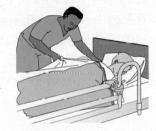

Fig. 9-49.

19 Ask your loved one to turn onto his back. Keep him covered and comfortable, with a pillow under his head.

20 Unfold the top sheet and place it over him. Ask him to hold the top sheet. Slip the blanket or old sheet out from underneath and put it in the hamper (Fig. 9-50).

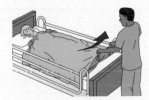

Fig. 9-50.

21 Place a blanket over the top sheet, matching the top edges. Tuck the bottom edges of top sheet and blanket under the bottom of the mattress, making square corners on each side. Loosen the top linens over the feet to prevent pressure. At the top of the bed, fold the top sheet over the blanket about six inches.

22 Remove the pillow. Do not hold it near your face. Remove the soiled pillowcase by turning it inside out and place it in the hamper. Remove your gloves.

23 With one hand, grasp the clean pillowcase at the closed end and turn it inside out over your arm. Using the hand with the pillowcase over it, grasp one narrow edge of the pillow and pull the pillowcase over it with your free hand (Fig. 9-51). Do the same with the other pillow. Place them as your loved one desires.

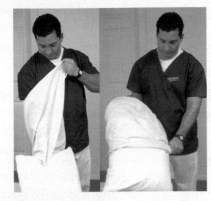

Fig. 9-51.

24 If you raised an adjustable bed, return it to its lowest position.

25 Put any signaling device within reach.

26 Wash your hands.

Making an unoccupied bed

Equipment: *clean linen: mattress pad, fitted or flat bottom sheet, waterproof bed protector if needed, blanket(s), cotton draw sheet, flat top sheet, pillowcase(s), gloves (if you're going to be touching linens soiled with body fluids)*

1 Wash your hands.

2 Discuss what you will do.

3 Provide privacy.

4 If bed is adjustable, adjust it to a safe working level, usually waist high. If bed is movable, lock bed wheels.

5	Put on gloves if you will be touching linens that are soiled with body fluids.
6	Loosen soiled linen. Roll soiled linen (soiled side inside) from head to foot of bed. Avoid contact with your skin or clothes. Place it in a hamper/bag, at foot of the bed, or in chair. Remove your gloves.
7	Remake the bed, spreading mattress pad and bottom sheet, tucking under. Make hospital corners to keep bottom sheet wrinkle-free. Put on mattress protector and draw sheet, smooth, and tuck under sides of bed.
8	Place top sheet and blanket over bed. Center, tuck under end of bed, and make hospital corners. Fold down the top sheet over the blanket about six inches. Fold both top sheet and blanket down so your loved one can easily get into bed. If he will not be returning to bed immediately, leave bedding up.
9	Remove pillows and pillowcases. Remove gloves. Put on clean pillowcases as described in procedure above. Replace pillows.
10	If you raised an adjustable bed, return it to its lowest position.
11	Put signaling device with reach.
12	Wash hands.

Resources

Abledata, sponsored by the National Institute on Disability and Rehabilitation Research (NIDRR), provides objective reviews of assistive devices and technology. They do not sell the products they review, but provide links to sites where they can be purchased.

ABLEDATA
8630 Fenton Street, Suite 930
Silver Spring, MD 20910
Tel: 800-227-0216
Fax: 301-608-8958
TT: 301-608-8912
www.abledata.com

Monterey Network of Care is an Internet-based network offering resources to caregivers, consumers and service providers.

Monterey Network of Care
Trilogy Integrated Resources LLC
1101 Fifth Ave., Suite 250
San Rafael, CA 94901
www.monterey.networkofcare.org

10

Transfers and Ambulation: Helping Your Loved One Get Around

As a family caregiver, you may often find yourself helping your loved one to stand, walk, move from a chair or bed, and stay steady on her feet. This can put tremendous physical strain on you; it can even be dangerous for both you and your loved one if done improperly. Learning to assist with changing positions and getting around, or transfers and ambulation, will make life safer and more comfortable for you both.

First Steps

Before moving your loved one into your home, make sure that you have the strength to assist him with ambulation and positioning if necessary, or that you will have other people or assistive devices to help you.

Have a healthcare professional demonstrate the procedures that you will be using to make sure that you are able to do them correctly. Whenever changes in your loved one's condition require you to learn a new procedure, ask a professional to demonstrate it for you.

Assess your loved one's mobility needs. Would he benefit from adaptive devices such as a cane or walker? If he already uses adaptive devices, are they in good working order? Is he using them properly?

Lifting, Holding, or Transferring Your Loved One

Review the principles of body mechanics in chapter 4. Always use good body mechanics when moving or positioning your loved one. Avoid lifting whenever possible; instead, push, roll, slide, or pivot, so that you are bearing less weight. Using good body mechanics will help protect you both from injury.

Before a person who has been lying down moves to a standing position, she should dangle, or sit up with her feet over the side of the bed, for a moment to regain her equilibrium, or bal-

ance. If your loved one is unable to walk, simply sitting up and dangling her legs may be ordered as part of a daily routine.

Assisting a person to a dangling position

1	Wash your hands.
2	Discuss what you will do.
3	Provide privacy as needed.
4	If the bed is adjustable, position it at lowest position. If the bed is movable, lock bed wheels.
5	Raise the head of the bed to the sitting position.
6	Place one arm under your loved one's shoulder blades and place the other arm under her thighs. (Fig. 10-1).
7	On the count of three, slowly turn her into a sitting position with legs dangling over the side of the bed (Fig. 10-2).
8	Ask her to hold onto the edge of the mattress with both hands. Assist her to put on non-skid shoes or slippers.
9	Have her dangle as long as ordered. Stay with her at all times. Check her for dizziness; if she feels dizzy or faint, help her lie down again. Report this to the doctor. This can

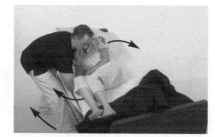

Fig. 10-1.

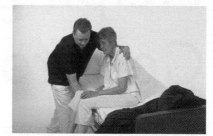

Fig. 10-2.

be a good time to note vital signs like pulse and respirations if you are keeping track of them.

10 If returning your loved one to bed rather than preparing to walk or transfer, remove her slippers or shoes.

11 Gently assist her back to bed. Place one arm around her shoulders and the other arm under her knees. Slowly swing her legs onto the bed.

12 Make sure she is comfortable.

13 Wash your hands after your loved one is safely back in bed or the transfer is completed.

14 Note what you did and any observations. How did she tolerate sitting up? Did she become dizzy?

Helping someone sit up using the arm lock

1 Wash your hands.

2 Discuss what you will do.

3 Provide privacy as needed.

4 If the bed is adjustable, adjust it to a safe level, usually waist high. If the bed is movable, lock bed wheels.

5 Stand facing the head of the bed, with your legs about 12 inches apart and your knees bent. The foot that is further from the bed should be slightly ahead of the other foot (Fig. 10-3).

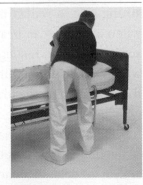

Fig. 10-3.

6 Place your arm under her armpit and grasp her shoulder. Have her grasp your shoulder in the same manner. This hold is called the armlock or lock arm (Fig. 10-4).

7 Reach under her head and place your other hand on her far shoulder. Have her bend her knees. Bend your knees.

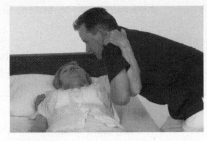

Fig. 10-4.

8 At the count of three, rock yourself backward and pull her to a sitting position. Use pillows or a bed rest to support her in the sitting position.

9 Check her for dizziness or weakness.

10 If you raised an adjustable bed, return it to its proper position.

11 Wash your hands.

12 Note any observations. Was she able to help at all? Did she become dizzy?

Helping someone stand up

1 Wash your hands.

2 Discuss what you will do.

3 Provide privacy as needed.

4 If the bed is adjustable, adjust it to a safe level, usually waist high. If the bed is movable, lock bed wheels.

5 Assist your loved one to a dangling position (see first procedure in this chapter).

6 Assist her to put on non-skid shoes or slippers.

7 If she is able, have her place her hands on the edge of the

bed and push to stand. Stay nearby to steady her or offer support if needed.

8	Always allow her to do whatever she is able to do for herself. If she is not able to stand without help, place one foot between her feet. If she has a weak knee, brace it against your knee (Fig. 10-5).
9	Have your loved one place her stronger leg directly underneath herself.
10	Bending your knees and leaning forward, put both arms around her waist and hold her close to your center of gravity (Fig. 10-6).
11	Tell her to lean forward, push down on the bed with her hands, and stand on the count of three. When you start to count, begin to rock. At three, rock your weight onto your back foot and assist her to a standing position.
12	Check your loved one for dizziness before you allow her to stand alone. If you raised an adjustable bed, return it to its proper position.
13	Wash your hands.
14	Note any observations. How did she tolerate standing? How much help did you offer?

If at any time your loved one starts to fall, widen your stance

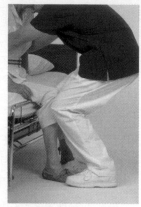

Fig. 10-5.

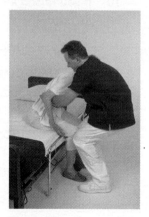

Fig. 10-6.

and bring her body close to you to break the fall. Bend your knees and support her as you lower her to the floor. You may need to drop to the floor yourself as you do this. Do not try to reverse or stop a fall; this can injure you and your loved one. Breaking the fall is the best and safest action to take.

If your loved one has fallen, call for help if anyone else is around. Do not try to get her up after the fall until you are certain she is not injured. Then get her into bed and report to the doctor. If you suspect that your loved one has been injured, do not move her. Call for emergency help immediately.

Adaptive Equipment

If your loved one uses a cane, crutches, or a walker, you should understand the purpose of each device (Fig. 10-7). The purpose of a cane is to assist with balance. A straight cane is not designed to bear weight. A quad cane, with four rubber-tipped feet, is designed to bear some weight. A person using any cane should be able to bear weight on both of his legs. If one leg is weaker, the cane should be held in the hand on the strong side. A walker is used when a person can bear some weight on his legs. The walker provides stability for those who are unsteady or who lack balance. The metal frame of the walker may have rubber-tipped feet and/or wheels. Crutches are used when a person can bear

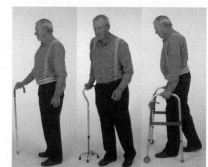

Cane   Quad cane   Walker

Fig. 10-7. If your loved one has difficulty walking, he may use a cane, crutches, or a walker.

no weight or limited weight on one leg; a person may use one crutch or two.

Whichever device is used, you can help ensure safety. Stay near the person, on his weak side. Make sure the equipment is in proper condition. It must be sturdy, and it must have rubber tips or wheels on the bottom.

A transfer belt, or gait belt, is used to assist those who are able to walk but are weak, unsteady, or uncoordinated. The belt is made of canvas or other heavy material and fits around the waist, outside the clothing. The transfer belt is a safety device that gives you something firm to hold on to. When placing the belt on your loved one, leave enough room to insert two fingers into the belt.

Using a transfer belt to assist with ambulation

1 Wash your hands.

2 Discuss what you will do.

3 Provide privacy as needed.

4 If the bed is adjustable, adjust it to a safe level, usually waist high. If the bed is movable, lock bed wheels.

5 Place the belt around your loved one's waist. Always apply the belt over clothing. *Never* place it next to skin.

6 Help him stand up, as described in earlier procedure. Observe him for strength and coordination.

7 Stand behind him and to his side as you hold on to the belt. If he has a weaker side, stand on that side. Use the hand that is not holding the belt to offer him support on the weak side (Fig. 10-8).

8 Observe his strength while you walk together. Provide a chair if he becomes dizzy or fatigued.

9 Return him to the bed or chair. Be sure he is positioned comfortably.

10 Wash your hands.

11 Note any observations. How far did he walk? How did he appear or say he felt while walking? How much help did you give?

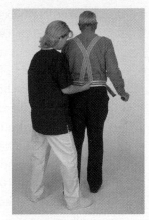
Fig. 10-8.

Assisting with walking for someone who uses a cane, walker, or crutches

1 Wash your hands.

2 Discuss what you will do.

3 Provide privacy as needed.

4 If the bed is adjustable, adjust it to a safe level, usually waist high. If the bed is movable, lock bed wheels.

5 Fasten the transfer belt around his waist.

6 Assist with putting on non-skid slippers or shoes.

7 Assist him to a standing position.

8 Assist as necessary with ambulation.

a **Cane**. Your loved one places the cane about 12 inches in front of his stronger leg. He brings the weaker leg even with the cane, and then brings the stronger leg forward slightly ahead of the cane (Fig. 10-9). He repeats these steps while ambulating.

Transfers and Ambulation

10

b **Walker**. He picks up or rolls the walker and places it about 12 inches in front of him. All four feet or wheels of the walker should be on the ground before he steps forward to the walker. The walker should not be moved again until he has moved both feet forward and is in a steady position (Fig. 10-10). He should never put his feet ahead of the walker.

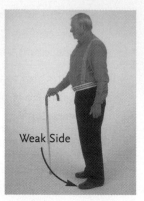

Weak Side

Fig. 10-9.

c **Crutches**. He should be fitted for crutches and taught to use them correctly by a physical therapist or nurse. He may use the crutches several different ways, depending on what his weakness is. No matter how he is using the crutches, weight should be on his hands and arms rather than on the underarm area (Fig. 10-11).

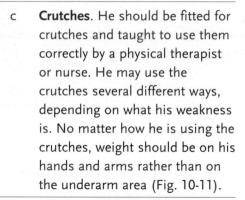

Fig. 10-10.

9 Whether he is using a cane, walker, or crutches, walk slightly behind him, on the weak side if he has one. Hold the transfer belt if one is used.

10 Watch for obstacles in his path, and encourage him to look ahead, rather than down at his feet.

11 Encourage him to rest if fatigued.

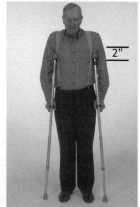

2"

Fig. 10-11.

When a person is fatigued, it increases the chance of a fall. Let him set the pace, and discuss how far he plans to go based on the physician's orders.

12 After ambulation, remove the transfer belt and help him into a safe and comfortable position.

13 If the bed was adjusted, return it to its proper position.

14 Wash your hands.

15 Note observations. How did he feel or appear while walking? How far did he walk? How much help did he need?

GUIDELINES
Wheelchairs

Learn how your loved one's wheelchair works, including how to apply and release the brake and how to operate the footrests. Always lock a wheelchair before assisting a person into or out of it (Fig. 10-12). After a transfer, unlock the wheelchair.

To transfer to or from a wheelchair, your loved one must use the side or areas of the body that can bear weight to support or lift the side or areas that cannot bear weight. If he can bear no weight with his legs, he may need to use leg braces or an overhead trapeze to support himself during a transfer.

The best thing you can do is make sure your loved one is safe and comfortable while

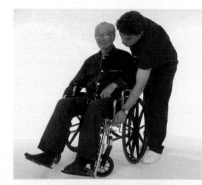

Fig. 10-12. You must always lock a wheelchair before your loved one gets into or out of it.

transferring to or from the wheelchair. Discuss how you can assist. You may only need to bring the chair to the bedside, or you may need to be more involved. Always be sure the chair is as close as possible to your loved one and that the chair is locked in place. Use a transfer belt if you are going to assist in the transfer. Be sure the transfer is done slowly, allowing time for your loved one to rest. Check his body alignment in the chair when the transfer is complete.

If your loved one needs to be moved back in the seat of the wheelchair, go to the back of the chair and reach forward and down under his arms. Ask him to place his feet on the ground and push up. Pull him up in the chair while he pushes.

Helping someone move from a bed to a chair

Equipment: robe, non-skid footwear, transfer belt, chair or wheelchair, sheet or blanket

1   Wash your hands.

2   Discuss what you will do.

3   Provide privacy as needed. Check the area to be certain it is uncluttered and safe.

4   Assist your loved one to the dangling position, as in earlier procedure.

5   Place the chair or wheelchair at the side of the bed on your loved one's stronger side. The chair should be at an angle slightly facing him. If using a wheelchair, lock the brakes and raise or remove the foot and leg rests so they are not in the way. Cover plastic seats with a bath blanket or a soft pillow.

6   Help him stand up, as in earlier procedure (Fig. 10-13).

7   Ask him to take small steps in the direction of the chair while turning his back toward the chair. If more assistance is needed, have him pivot on the foot that is further away from the chair. Always allow him to do all he can for himself.

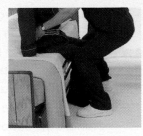

Fig. 10-13.

8   Have him use one arm to grasp the arm of the chair. When the chair is touching the back of his legs, help him lower himself into the chair.

9   If using a wheelchair, lower the footrests and help him place his feet on them. Check that he is in good alignment. Place a lap robe, folded blanket, or sheet over the lap as appropriate.

10   Wash your hands.

11   Note any observations. How did your loved one feel or appear during the transfer? How much assistance was required?

A slide board may be used to help transfer someone who is unable to bear weight on her legs. Slide boards can be used for almost any transfer that involves moving from one sitting or reclining position to another. For example, slide boards can be helpful for transfers from bed to chair, from wheelchair to bathtub, and from wheelchair to car.

Helping someone transfer using a slide board

1   Follow steps 1 through 5 of the procedure for helping someone move from a bed to a chair (above).

2   Have your loved one lean away from transfer side to take the weight off her thigh (Fig. 10-14). Place one end of the slide board under the buttocks and thigh, taking care not to pinch her skin be-

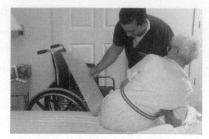

Fig. 10-14.

tween the bed and the board. Place the other end of the sliding board on the surface to which she is transferring.

3   If she is able, have your loved one push up with her hands and scoot herself across the board. Stay close so you can provide support if needed. Always allow her to do all she can for herself.

4   If she needs assistance, stand in front of her and put your knees in front and a little to the outside of her knees to keep them from buckling during the transfer. Make sure your back is straight.

5   Get as close to her as possible and have her lean into you as you grasp the transfer belt from behind. Lean back with your knees bent. Using your legs rather than your back, pull her up slightly and toward you to help her scoot across the board (Fig. 10-15).

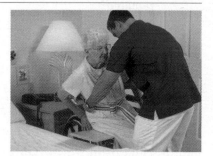

Fig. 10-15.

6   Complete the transfer in two or three lifting and scooting movements. *Never* drag her across the board. Friction

from the skin dragging across the slide board can cause skin breakdown that can lead to pressure sores.

7   After your loved one is safely transferred, remove the slide board. Make sure she is positioned safely and comfortably.

8   Wash your hands.

9   Note any observations. How did she feel or appear during the transfer? How much assistance was required?

You may have a mechanical lift in the home. There are various types of mechanical and hydraulic lifts; you must be trained to use the specific lift in your home (Fig. 10-16). Contact the physical or occupational therapist and follow the manufacturer's instructions whenever using the lift.

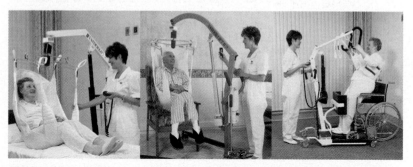

Fig. 10-16. Today, there are lifts that transfer completely dependent people and people who can bear some weight. (Photos courtesy of VANCARE Inc., 800-694-4525)

Transferring someone using a mechanical lift

Equipment: wheelchair or chair, lifting partner (if available), mechanical or hydraulic lift

1   Wash your hands.

2   Discuss what you will do. Ask someone to help you.

3   Provide privacy as needed.

4   If bed is movable, lock bed wheels.

5   Position wheelchair next to bed. Lock brakes.

6   Help your loved one turn to one side of the bed. Position the sling under her, with the edge next to her back fanfolded if necessary. Fanfolding means folding several times into pleats. Make the bottom of the sling even with her knees. Help her roll back to the middle of the bed, and then spread out the fanfolded edge of the sling.

7   Roll the mechanical lift to bedside. Make sure the base is opened to its widest point, and push the base of the lift under the bed.

8   Position the overhead bar directly over her (Fig. 10-17).

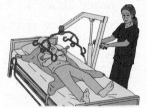

Fig. 10-17.

9   With your loved one lying on her back, attach one set of straps to each side of the sling and one set of straps to the overhead bar (Fig. 10-18). If a lifting partner is available, have him support your loved one at the head, shoulders, and knees while she is being lifted. Her arms should be folded across her chest (Fig. 10-19). If the device has "S" hooks, they should face away from her (Fig. 10-20). Make sure all straps are connected properly.

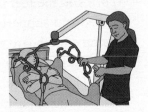

Fig. 10-18.

10   Following manufacturer's instructions, raise her two inches above the bed. Pause for a moment for her to gain equilibrium.

11   If a lifting partner is available, he can help support and guide your loved one while you roll the lift so that she is positioned over the chair or wheelchair.

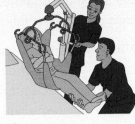

Fig. 10-19.

12   Slowly lower her into the chair or wheelchair. Push down gently on her knees to help her into a sitting position.

13   Undo the straps from the overhead bar to the sling. Leave the sling in place for transfer back to the bed.

14   Be sure your loved one is seated comfortably and correctly in the chair or wheelchair.

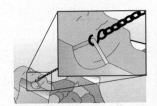

Fig. 10-20.

15   Wash your hands.

16   Note any observations. How did she tolerate the transfer? Were there any problems during the transfer? Did the equipment operate properly?

Positioning

Five Basic Positions

A person who spends a lot of time in bed often needs help getting into a comfortable position. She also needs to change positions frequently to avoid skin breakdown or pressure sores. Positioning means helping a person into positions that will be comfortable and healthy. If your loved one is bed-bound, she should be repositioned every two hours. The position and time should be documented every time there is a change, so a 24-hour plan can be followed.

Which positions are used will depend upon your loved one's diagnosis, her condition, and her preferences. Even if she cannot move herself voluntarily, she may not stay in the position you put her in, so you will need to check her position periodically. Keep body mechanics and alignment in mind when positioning. Also, check skin for blanching (turning white) or redness, especially around bony areas, each time you reposition.

The following are guidelines for positioning your loved one in the five basic body positions:

1. **Supine**: In this position, your loved one is lying flat on his back. To maintain correct body position, support his head and shoulders with a pillow (Fig. 10-21). You may also use pillows, rolled towels, or washcloths to support his arms (especially a weak or immobilized arm) or hands. The heels should be "floating." This is done by placing a very firm pillow under the calves so the heels do not touch the bed. Pillows or a footboard can be used to keep feet flexed slightly.

2. **Lateral/side**: A person in the lateral position is lying on either side of his body. There are many variations of the lateral, or side, position. Pillows can support the arm and leg on the upper side, the back, and the head (Fig. 10-22). Ideally, the knee

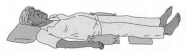

Fig. 10-21. A person in the supine position is flat on her back.

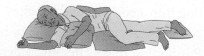

Fig. 10-22. A person in the lateral position is lying on his side.

on the upper side of the body should be flexed, with the leg brought in front of the body and supported on a pillow. There should be a pillow under the bottom foot so that the toes are not touching the bed. If the top leg cannot be brought forward and instead rests on the bottom leg, pillows should be used between the two legs to relieve pressure and avoid skin breakdown.

3. **Prone**: A person in the prone position is lying on her stomach, or the front side of her body (Fig. 10-23). This is not a comfortable position for many people, especially elderly people. Use the prone position with care and only for short periods. In this position, the arms are either at the sides or raised above the head. The head is turned to one side and a small pillow may be used under the head.

4. **Fowler's**: A person in Fowler's position is in a semi-sitting position, with the head and shoulders elevated (Fig. 10-24). Her knees may be flexed and elevated using a pillow or rolled blanket as a support, and the feet may be flexed and supported using a footboard or other support. The spine should be straight. In a true Fowler's position the upper body is raised to a point halfway between sitting straight up and lying flat. In a semi-Fowler's position the upper body is not raised as high.

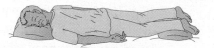

Fig. 10-23. A person in the prone position is lying on his stomach.

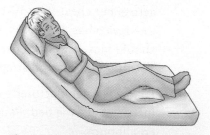

Fig. 10-24. A person in Fowler's position is partially reclined.

5. **Sims':** The Sims' position is a variation on the lateral, or side, position. It is a left side-lying position. The lower arm is behind the back. The upper knee is flexed and raised toward the chest,

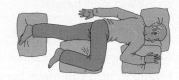

Fig. 10-25. A person in Sims' position is lying on his side with one leg drawn up.

using a pillow as a support (Fig. 10-25). There should be a pillow under the bottom foot so that the toes do not touch the bed.

Use the positions that the doctor, nurse, or physical therapist recommends for your loved one. In general, these should be positions that are natural and comfortable for him. Always remember to check the skin for signs of irritation whenever you reposition.

Turning someone in bed

1 Wash your hands.

2 Discuss what you will do.

3 Provide privacy as needed.

4 If the bed is adjustable, adjust bed to a safe level, usually waist high. If bed is movable, lock bed wheels.

5 With your loved one in supine position and centered in the bed, stand at the side of the bed she will face. Place her near hand palm up under her hip.

6 Lift her far leg over her near leg, flexing the knee (Fig. 10-26).

7 Assume a good stance: your feet hip width apart, your

knees bent, and one foot slightly in front of the other.

8 Grasp her far shoulder and far hip. Count to three, rocking your weight forward and back on each count. On three, roll her onto her side (Fig. 10-27).

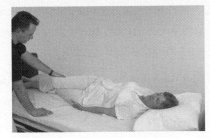

Fig. 10-26.

9 Use pillows or supports as necessary to be sure she is in a comfortable position with good body alignment. Arrange the bed covers so that she is comfortable. If you raised an adjustable bed, return it to its proper position.

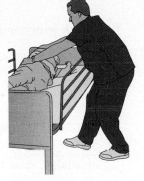

10 Wash your hands.

Fig. 10-27.

11 Note any observations.

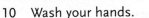

Helping your loved one move up in bed helps prevent skin irritation that can lead to pressure sores. It is best to have a helper assist you. If you must do it by yourself and your loved one cannot help, use a draw sheet or turning sheet (Fig. 10-28). A draw sheet is an extra sheet placed over the bottom sheet when the bed is made. It allows you to reposi-

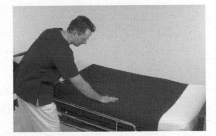

Fig. 10-28. A draw sheet is used to move a person in bed without causing shearing of the skin.

tion the person in bed without causing shearing, or friction and pressure on the skin from rubbing or dragging it across a surface (the bottom sheet).

Always allow your loved one to do all she can for herself. Following is the procedure for someone who can help you move her up in bed.

Moving someone up in bed

1	Wash your hands.
2	Discuss what you will do.
3	Provide privacy as needed.
4	If the bed is adjustable, adjust it to a safe working level, usually waist high. Lower the head of the bed to make it flat. If the bed is movable, lock bed wheels. If side rails are available, raise the rail on the far side of the bed. Remove the pillow and set it aside for later use.
5	Place one arm under your loved one's shoulders and the other under her buttocks.
6	Ask her to bend her knees and push down on the mattress with her feet and hands on the count of three (Fig. 10-29).
7	Keeping your back straight and bending at the knees, help her move toward the head of the mattress on the count of three.

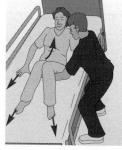

Fig. 10-29.

8	Help her into a comfortable position and arrange the pillow and blankets for her. If you raised an adjustable bed, be sure to return it to its proper position.

9	Wash your hands.
10	Note any observations.

When your loved one cannot assist and there is no one else around to help you move her up in bed, take the following steps:

1	Follow steps 1 through 3 above.
2	If the bed is adjustable, adjust it to a safe working level, usually waist high. Lower the head of the bed to make it flat. If the bed is movable, lock bed wheels. Raise both side rails if side rails are available.
3	Stand behind the head of the bed with your feet shoulder width apart and one foot slightly in front of the other.
4	Roll and grasp the top edge of the draw sheet.
5	With your knees bent and your back straight, rock your weight from the front foot to the back foot in one smooth motion (Fig. 10-30).

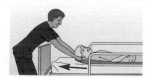

Fig. 10-30.

6	Help your loved one into a comfortable position and arrange the pillow and blankets for her. Unroll the draw sheet and leave it in place for the next repositioning. If you raised an adjustable bed, be sure to return it to its proper position.
7	Wash your hands.
8	Note any observations.

When you have help from another person, you can modify the procedure as follows:

1	Follow steps 1 through 3 from above.

2   If the bed is adjustable, adjust it to a safe working level, usually waist high. Lower the head of the bed to make it flat. If the bed is movable, lock bed wheels.

3   Stand on the opposite side of the bed from your helper. Each of you should be turned slightly toward the head of the bed. For each of you, the foot that is closest to the head of the bed should be pointed in that direction.

4   Roll the draw sheet up to your loved one's side; have your helper do the same on his side of the bed. Grasp the sheet with your palms up, and have your helper do the same.

5   Shift your weight to your back foot (the foot closer to the foot of the bed) and have your helper do the same (Fig. 10-31). On the count of three, you and your helper both shift your weight to your forward feet as you slide the draw sheet toward the head of the bed (Fig. 10-32).

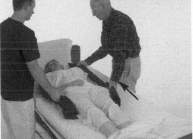
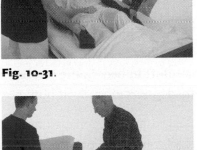

Fig. 10-31.

Fig. 10-32.

6   Help your loved one into a comfortable position and arrange the pillow and blankets for her. Unroll the draw sheet and leave it in place for the next repositioning.

7   If you raised an adjustable bed, be sure to return it to its proper position.

8   Wash your hands.

9   Note any observations.

Sometimes the spinal column must be kept in alignment. To turn a person in bed while maintaining alignment of the spine, you will use a procedure called logrolling.

Logrolling a person

1   Wash your hands.

2   Discuss what you will do.

3   Provide privacy as needed.

4   If the bed is adjustable, adjust it to a safe working level, usually waist high. Lower the head of the bed to make it flat. If the bed is movable, lock bed wheels.

5   Move your loved one to the side of the bed you are standing on. To do this, assume a good stance, with feet hip width apart, knees bent, and one foot slightly in front of the other. Slip your arms under her shoulders and move her toward you by rocking your weight backward onto your back foot (Fig. 10-33). Keep your knees bent. Be careful not to slide her across the sheets and cause shearing (pressure on the skin from sliding across another surface), which can lead to pressure sores.

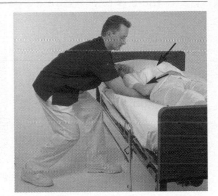

Fig. 10-33.

6   Keeping the same good stance, slide your arms under her hips and shift them toward you as you did her shoulders (Fig. 10-34). Make sure her head and legs are in alignment with her shoulders and hips before continuing with the procedure.

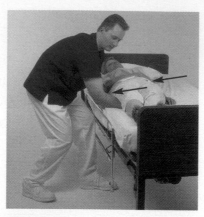

Fig. 10-34.

7   If available, raise the side rail on the side of the bed she is now closest to. If no side rail is available, be sure she is safe and stable before moving to the next step.

8   Move to the other side of the bed and lower the side rail if there is one. Assume a good stance.

9   With your knees bent, grasp her with one hand on the far hip and one on the far shoulder. Roll her toward you onto her side (Fig. 10-35).

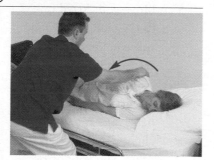

Fig. 10-35.

10 Check her body alignment. Arrange pillows and covers for comfort. Raise the side rail if available and if necessary for safety. If you raised an adjustable bed, be sure to return it to its proper position.

11 Wash your hands.

12 Note any observations.

Comfort Measures

The following are some ideas to help enhance your loved one's comfort and safety in and around the bed:

- Have plenty of pillows available to provide support in various positions.

- Use positioning devices (such as backrests, bed cradles and tables, footboards, and handrolls—details on these devices follow).

- Give backrubs for comfort and relaxation.

- Change her position frequently, at least every two hours or as directed.

- Always maintain body alignment.

Many positioning devices are available to help promote comfort in bed. Some can be made inexpensively at home.

Backrests can be made of pillows, cardboard or wood covered by pillows, or special wedge-shaped foam pillows (Fig. 10-36).

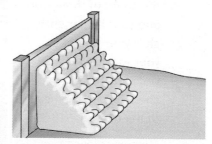

Fig. 10-36. A backrest.

Bed cradles are used to keep the bed covers from pushing down on the feet. Metal frames that work like a tent when the bed covers are over them can be purchased at

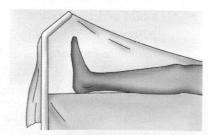

Fig. 10-37. A bed cradle.

medical supply stores (Fig. 10-37). A cardboard box can be used as a bed cradle by placing the feet inside the box underneath the covers (Fig. 10-38). The box should be at least two inches above the toes.

Bed tables are available commercially, or you can make one by cutting openings in each of the longer sides of a sturdy cardboard box (Fig. 10-39).

Draw sheets or turning sheets may be placed under your loved one and used to help move her if she is unable to assist with turning in bed, lifting, or moving up in bed. A regular bed sheet folded in half can be used as a draw sheet.

Footboards are padded boards placed against the feet to keep them flexed and to prevent footdrop (Fig. 10-40). Rolled blankets or pillows can also be used as footboards.

Handrolls keep the fingers from curling tightly. A rolled washcloth, gauze bandage, or a rubber ball placed inside the palm

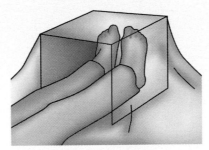

Fig. 10-38. A homemade bed cradle.

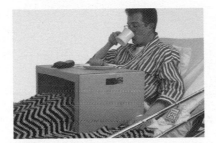

Fig. 10-39. A bed table.

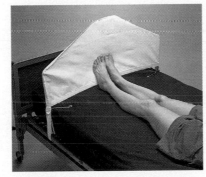

Fig. 10-40. A footboard. (Reprinted with permission of Briggs Corporation, 800-247-2343)

may be used to keep the hand in a natural position (Fig. 10-41).

Splints may be prescribed to keep your loved one's joints in the correct position (Fig. 10-42).

Trochanter rolls are used to keep the hips from turning outward. A rolled towel works well as an improvised trochanter roll (Fig. 10-43).

Physical Restraints

Throughout this book, the safety of your loved one in the home has been the top priority. In the past, physical restraints, including vests and belts designed to restrict movement, were used in home care to safeguard patients who wandered, were violent, or were at risk of hurting themselves. However, because overuse and abuse of these restraints became common, many states now restrict their use. In some states restraints are illegal. In oth-

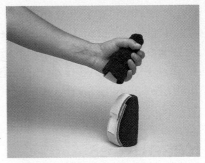

Fig. 10-41. A handroll. (Reprinted with permission of Briggs Corporation, 800-247-2343)

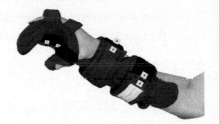

Fig. 10-42. One type of splint. (Photo courtesy of Lenjoy Medical Engineering, 800-582-5332, www.comfysplints.com)

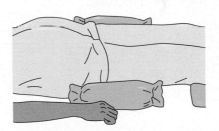

Fig. 10-43. Trochanter rolls.

ers, restraints may only be used for specified periods of time. If you are concerned for the safety of your loved one because he is wandering or becoming aggressive or violent, you must discuss this with your doctor. There may be safer ways to manage this behavior in the home.

Resources

Abledata, sponsored by the National Institute on Disability and Rehabilitation Research (NIDRR), provides objective reviews of assistive devices and technology. They do not sell the products they review, but provide links to sites where they can be purchased.

ABLEDATA
8630 Fenton Street, Suite 930
Silver Spring, MD 20910
Tel: 800-227-0216
Fax: 301-608-8958
TT: 301-608-8912
Email: abledata@orcmacro.com
www.abledata.com

Basic Healthcare Skills

As mentioned previously, much of the material in this book was originally developed to train home health aides, who provide essential nursing care in the home. As a family caregiver, you may wish to become familiar with this training in essential nursing skills, either to better monitor care your loved one receives from others or for your own use. In this chapter we describe the correct methods for observing and recording vital signs, collecting specimens, and various other special procedures that your loved one may require. Always check with the doctor and other members of the care team to find out which procedures are appropriate for you to perform.

First Steps

Ask a professional healthcare provider, such as a physician or nurse, to show you how to perform the procedures listed in the chapter. Make sure you are shown any specific adaptations that need to be made for your loved one's condition.

Make sure that you have all of the supplies listed for the procedures you will be performing, including equipment for monitoring vital signs and any necessary personal protective equipment (see chapter 5).

Be aware of the normal levels for all of the vital signs you will be monitoring. Know what is normal for your loved one and what should prompt you to call the physician.

Vital Signs

Vital signs show how well the vital organs of the body, such as the heart and lungs, are working. They consist of the following:

- body temperature
- pulse
- rate of respirations (breaths)
- blood pressure
- level of pain

Watching for changes in vital signs is important. They can indicate when your loved one's condition is changing or worsening. Always notify the doctor if your loved one:

- is running a fever
- has a respiratory (breathing) or pulse rate that is too rapid or too slow
- has a change in blood pressure
- has pain that is worse or that is not relieved by pain management

Normal Ranges for Adult Vital Signs

Temperature:	Fahrenheit	Celsius
Oral (mouth)	97.6°- 99.6°	36.5°- 37.5°
Rectal (rectum)	98.6°- 100.6°	37.0°- 38.1°
Axillary (underarm)	96.6°- 98.6°	36.0°- 37.0°

Pulse: 60-90 beats per minute

Respirations: 12-20 respirations per minute

Blood Pressure:

Normal: Systolic 100-119, Diastolic 60-79

Prehypertension: Systolic 120-139, Diastolic 80-89

High: 140/90 or above *

* Millions of people whose blood pressure was previously considered normal (120/80) now fall into the "prehypertension" range. Prehypertension means that the person does not have high blood pressure now but is likely to develop it in the future. This is based on the new, more aggressive high blood pressure guidelines from the Seventh Report of the Joint National Committee (JNC 7) on Prevention, Detection, Evaluation and Treatment of High Blood Pressure (2003).

Temperature

Body temperature is normally very close to 98.6° F (Fahrenheit) or 37° C (Celsius). Body temperature reflects a balance between the heat created by our bodies and the heat lost to the environment. Increases in body temperature may indicate an infection or disease. There are four sites for taking body temperature:

1. the mouth (oral)

2. the rectum (rectal)

3. the armpit (axillary)

4. the ear (tympanic)

The different sites require different types of thermometers. The site you use will depend on what kind of thermometer is available. There is a range of normal temperatures. Some people's temperatures normally run low; others in completely good health will run slightly higher temperatures. Normal temperature readings also vary by the method used to take the temperature. A rectal temperature is generally considered to be the most accurate; axillary temperature is considered the least accurate.

Temperatures are most often taken orally. Do not take an oral temperature on a person who:

- is unconscious

- is using oxygen

- is confused or disoriented

- is paralyzed from stroke

- has facial trauma

- is younger than six years old

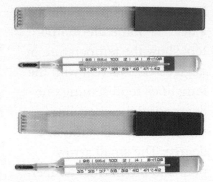

Fig. 11-1. A mercury-free oral thermometer and a mercury-free rectal thermometer (Photos provided by RG Medical Diagnostics of Southfield, MI.)

Using glass bulb or mercury thermometers to take oral or rectal temperatures used to be common. However, because mercury is a dangerous, toxic substance, many states have passed laws to ban the sale of mercury thermometers.

Mercury-free thermometers are becoming more common (Fig. 11-1). They can be used to take an oral or rectal temperature, and they are considered much safer. Mercury-free thermometers can usually be purchased at your local pharmacy. If you are still using a mercury thermometer in your home, consider replacing it with a mercury-free thermometer. If you must use a mercury thermometer, be careful. If you break a glass thermometer, never touch the mercury or broken glass. Call your state pollution control agency or local health department to learn how to dispose of it properly.

Although mercury-free thermometers are slightly larger than glass-bulb thermometers, they operate identically. Numbers on the thermometer let you read the temperature after it registers. Most thermometers show the temperature in degrees Fahrenheit (F). Each long line represents one degree and each short

Basic Healthcare Skills

11

line represents two-tenths of a degree. Some thermometers show the temperature in degrees Celsius (C), with the long lines representing one degree and the short lines representing one-tenth of a degree. The small arrow points to the normal temperature: 98.6° F and 37° C (Fig. 11-2).

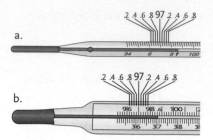

Fig. 11-2. A mercury glass thermometer (a) is read the same way as a mercury-free thermometer (b).

Battery-powered, digital, or electronic thermometers are other types of thermometers (Fig. 11-3). These thermometers display the results digitally and register the temperature more quickly than mercury-free or glass bulb thermometers. Digital thermometers usually take two to sixty seconds to register the temperature. The thermometer will beep or flash when the temperature has registered. Digital thermometers may be used to take oral, rectal, or axillary temperatures. Follow the manufacturer's guide for proper use of these thermometers.

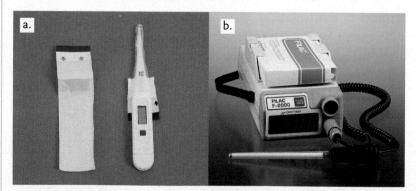

Fig. 11-3. a. A digital thermometer and b. an electronic thermometer.

The tympanic thermometer, or ear thermometer, also registers a temperature quickly (Fig. 11-4). However, these thermometers are expensive and may not be as common in the home. They also require more practice to be able to take accurate temperatures.

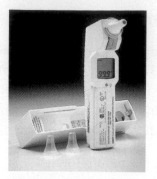

Fig. 11-4. A tympanic thermometer.

Taking and recording an oral temperature

Equipment: *mercury-free, glass, digital, or electronic thermometer; disposable plastic sheaths/covers for thermometers; tissues; pen and paper to record your findings*

Do not take an oral temperature if your loved one has smoked, eaten food or drunk fluids, or exercised in the last 10–20 minutes.

1 Wash your hands.

2 Discuss what you will do.

3 Provide privacy.

Using a mercury-free thermometer or glass thermometer:

4 Hold the thermometer by the stem.

5 Before inserting oral thermometer in the mouth, shake oral thermometer down to below the lowest number (at least below 96° F or 35° C). To shake the thermometer down, hold it at the side opposite the bulb with the thumb and two fingers. With a snapping motion of the wrist, shake the thermometer (Fig. 11-5). Stand away from furni-

ture and walls while doing this.

6   Put disposable sheath on the thermometer, if available. Insert the fluted tip or bulb end of oral thermometer into the mouth, under the tongue and to one side (Fig. 11-6).

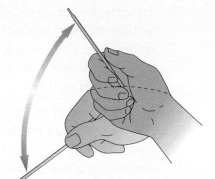

Fig. 11-5.

7   Tell your loved one to hold the thermometer in her mouth with her lips closed. Assist as necessary. She should breathe through her nose. Ask her not to bite down or to talk.

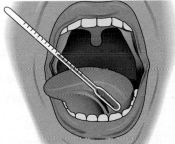
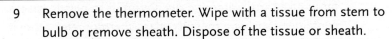

Fig. 11-6.

8   Leave the thermometer in place for at least three minutes. More time may be required if she opens her mouth to breathe or talk.

9   Remove the thermometer. Wipe with a tissue from stem to bulb or remove sheath. Dispose of the tissue or sheath.

10 Hold thermometer at eye level. Rotate until line appears, rolling the thermometer between your thumb and forefinger. Read and record temperature. Document the temperature, date, time and method used (oral).

Using a digital thermometer:

4   Put on disposable sheath if available.

5   Turn on thermometer and wait until "ready" sign appears.

6   Insert end of digital thermometer into the mouth, under tongue and to one side.

7   Leave in place until thermometer blinks or beeps.

8   Remove the thermometer.

9   Read and record temperature on display screen. Document the temperature, date, time and method used (oral).

10 Using a tissue, remove and dispose of sheath.

Using an electronic thermometer:

4   Remove probe from base unit.

5   Put on probe cover.

6   Insert end of electronic thermometer into the mouth, under tongue and to one side.

7   Leave in place until you hear a tone or see a flashing or steady light.

8   Read the temperature on the display screen.

9   Remove the probe. Press the eject button to discard the cover (Fig. 11-7).

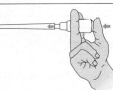

10 Document the temperature, date, time and method used (oral).

Fig. 11-7.

Final steps:

11 **Mercury-free, glass, or digital thermometer:** Rinse the thermometer in lukewarm water and dry. Return it to its plastic case or container. If using a mercury/glass thermometer, store it away from a heat source.

Electronic thermometer: Return the probe to the holder.

12 Wash your hands.

Taking and recording a rectal temperature

Equipment: rectal mercury-free, glass, or digital thermometer, lubricant, gloves, tissue, disposable plastic sheath/cover, pen and paper

1   Wash your hands.

2   Discuss what you will do.

3   Provide privacy.

4   Assist your loved one to the left-lying position (Fig. 11-8).

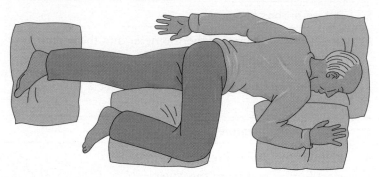

Fig. 11-8.

5   Fold back the linens to expose only the rectal area.

6   Put on gloves.

7   **Mercury-free or glass thermometer:** Hold thermometer by stem.

    Digital thermometer: Apply probe cover if available.

8   **Mercury-free or glass thermometer:** Shake the thermometer down to below the lowest number.

9   Apply a small amount of lubricant to tip or bulb or probe cover.

10 Separate the buttocks. Gently insert thermometer one inch into rectum (Fig. 11-9). Stop if you meet resistance. Do not force the thermometer in.

11 Replace the sheet over buttocks while holding onto the thermometer. Hold onto the thermometer at all times while taking a rectal temperature.

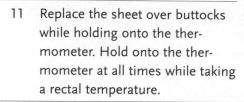

Fig. 11-9.

12 **Mercury-free or glass thermometer:** Hold thermometer in place for at least three minutes.

    Digital thermometer: Hold thermometer in place until thermometer blinks or beeps.

13 Gently remove the thermometer. Wipe with tissue from stem to bulb or remove sheath. Dispose of tissue or sheath.

14 Read the thermometer at eye level as you would for an oral temperature. Document the temperature, date, time and method used (rectal).

15 **Mercury-free or glass thermometer:** Rinse the thermometer in lukewarm water and dry. Return it to plastic case or container. If using a mercury/glass thermometer, store it away from a heat source.

    Digital thermometer: Throw away probe cover and store thermometer.

16 Remove and dispose of gloves.

17 Help your loved one return to a position that is safe and comfortable.

18 Wash your hands.

Taking and recording an axillary temperature

Equipment: *mercury-free, glass, digital, or electronic thermometer, tissues, disposable sheath/cover, pen and paper*

1   Wash your hands.

2   Discuss what you will do.

3   Provide privacy.

4   Adjust or remove enough of your loved one's clothing to allow skin contact with the end of the thermometer. Wipe axillary area with tissues to make sure it is dry before placing the thermometer under the arm.

Using a mercury-free thermometer or glass thermometer:

5   Hold the thermometer at the stem end. Shake down to below the lowest number.

6   Put disposable sheath on thermometer, if applicable.

7   Place bulb end of thermometer in center of the armpit. Fold arm over her chest.

8   Hold thermometer in place, with the arm close against the side, for 10 minutes (Fig. 11-10).

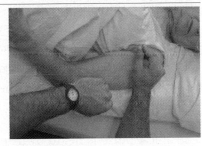

Fig. 11-10.

9   Remove the thermometer. Wipe with tissue from stem to bulb or remove sheath. Dispose of tissue or sheath.

10   Hold thermometer at eye level. Rotate until line appears. Read temperature. Document the temperature, date, time, and method used (axillary).

Using a digital thermometer:

5   Put on disposable sheath. Turn on thermometer and wait until "ready" sign appears.

6   Position end of digital thermometer in center of the armpit. Fold her arm over her chest.

7   Hold thermometer in place until it blinks or beeps.

8   Remove the thermometer.

9   Read the temperature on display screen. Record the temperature, date, time, and method used (axillary).

10   Using a tissue, remove and dispose of sheath.

Using an electronic thermometer:

5   Remove probe from base unit and put on probe cover.

6   Position the end of electronic thermometer in center of armpit. Fold her arm over her chest.

7   Leave thermometer in place until you hear a tone or see a flashing or steady light.

8   Read the temperature on the display screen.

9   Remove the probe and press the eject button to discard the cover.

10   Record the temperature, date, time, and method used (axillary).

Final steps:

11   **Mercury-free or glass thermometer:** Clean and store thermometer.

Digital thermometer: Replace thermometer in case.

Electronic thermometer: Return the probe to the holder.

12   Wash your hands.

Taking and recording a tympanic temperature

Equipment: tympanic thermometer, disposable probe sheath/cover, pen and paper

1   Wash your hands.

2   Discuss what you will do.

3   Provide privacy.

4   Put a disposable sheath over the earpiece of the thermometer.

5   Position your loved one's head so that the ear is in front of you. Straighten the ear canal by pulling up and back on the outside edge of the ear (Fig.11-11). Insert the covered probe into the ear canal and press the button.

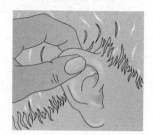

Fig. 11-11.

6   Hold thermometer in place until thermometer blinks or beeps.

7   Read the temperature. Record the temperature, date, time, and method used (tympanic).

8   Dispose of sheath. Put thermometer away.

9   Wash your hands.

Pulse

The pulse is the number of times a person's heart beats per minute. The beat that you feel at the pulse points in the body represents the wave of blood moving as a result of the heart pumping. The most common site for checking the pulse is on the inside of the wrist, where the radial artery runs just beneath the skin. This is called the radial pulse.

The brachial pulse is the pulse inside of the elbow, about 1–1½ inches above the elbow. The radial and brachial pulses are involved in taking blood pressure. Blood pressure is explained later in this chapter. Other common pulse sites are shown in Figure 11-12.

For adults, the normal pulse rate is 60–90 beats per minute. Small children have more rapid pulses, in the range of 100–120 beats per minute. A newborn baby's pulse may be as high as 120–140 beats per minute. Many things can affect pulse rate, including exercise, fear, anger, anxiety, heat, medications, and pain. An unusually high or low rate does not necessarily indicate disease; however, sometimes the pulse rate can signal serious illness. For example, a rapid pulse may result from fever, infection, or a heart condition. A slow or weak pulse may indicate dehydration, infection, or shock.

The apical pulse is heard by listening directly over the heart with a stethoscope. The apical pulse is on the left side of the chest, just below the nipple. For older adults, the apical pulse may be taken when the person has heart disease or takes drugs that affect the heart. It may also be taken on people who have a weak radial pulse or an irregular pulse.

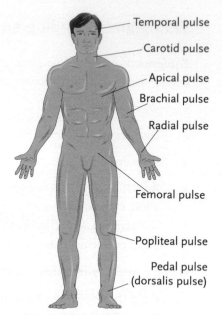

Temporal pulse
Carotid pulse
Apical pulse
Brachial pulse
Radial pulse
Femoral pulse
Popliteal pulse
Pedal pulse (dorsalis pulse)

Fig. 11-12. Common pulse sites.

Taking and recording apical pulse

Equipment: stethoscope, watch with second hand, alcohol wipes, pen and paper

1   Wash your hands.

2   Discuss what you will do.

3   Provide privacy as necessary.

4   Fit the earpieces of the stethoscope snugly in your ears. Place the flat metal diaphragm on the left side of the chest, just below the nipple (Fig. 11-13). Listen for the heartbeat.

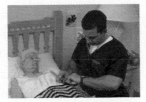

Fig. 11-13.

5   Using the second hand of your watch, count the heartbeats for one minute. Each "lub-dub" that you hear is counted as one beat. A normal heartbeat is rhythmical. Leave the stethoscope in place to count respirations (as described in the next procedure).

6   Document the pulse rate, date, time, and method used (apical). Note any irregularities in the rhythm.

7   Clean earpieces and diaphragm of stethoscope with alcohol wipes. Store stethoscope.

8   Wash your hands.

Respirations

Respiration is the process of breathing air into the lungs, or inspiration, and exhaling air out of the lungs, or expiration. Each respiration consists of an inspiration and an expiration. The chest rises during inspiration and falls during expiration.

The normal respiration rate for adults ranges from 12 to 20 breaths per minute. Infants and children have a faster respiratory rate. Infants can breathe normally at a rate of 30 to 40 respirations per minute. People may breathe more quickly if they know they are being observed. Because of this, count respirations immediately after taking the pulse. Keep your fingers on your loved one's wrist or the stethoscope over the heart. Do not make it obvious that you are observing her breathing.

Taking and recording radial pulse and counting and recording respirations

Equipment: watch with a second hand, pen and paper

1   Wash your hands.

2   Discuss what you will do.

3   Provide privacy.

4   Place fingertips on thumb side of the wrist to locate pulse (Fig. 11-14).

5   Count the beats for one full minute.

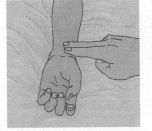

Fig. 11-14.

6   Keeping your fingertips on the wrist, count respirations for one full minute. Observe for the pattern and character of your loved one's breathing. Normal breathing is smooth and quiet. If you see signs of difficult breathing, shallow breathing, or noisy breathing, such as wheezing, report it to the doctor.

7   Document the pulse rate, date, time, and method used (radial). Notify the doctor if the pulse is less than 60 beats

per minute, over 90 beats per minute, or if the rhythm is irregular. Document the respiratory rate and the pattern or character of breathing.

8 Wash your hands.

Blood Pressure

Blood pressure is an important indicator of a person's health. Blood pressure is measured in millimeters of mercury (mmHg). The measurement shows how well the heart is working. There are two parts of blood pressure, the systolic measurement and diastolic measurement.

In the systolic phase, the heart is at work, contracting and pushing blood out of the left ventricle. The reading shows the pressure on the walls of the arteries as blood is pumped through the body. The normal range for systolic blood pressure is 100 to 119 mm Hg.

The second measurement reflects the diastolic phase—when the heart relaxes. The diastolic measurement is always lower than the systolic measurement. It shows the pressure in the arteries when the heart is at rest. The normal range for adults is 60 to 79 mm Hg.

People with high blood pressure, or hypertension, have elevated systolic and/or diastolic blood pressures. A blood pressure of 140/90 mmHg or higher is considered high.

However, if blood pressure is between 120/80 mmHg and 139/89 mmHg, it is called "prehypertension." This means that the person does not have high blood pressure now but is likely to develop it in the future. Report to your loved one's physician if his blood pressure is 140/90 or above.

Many factors can cause increased blood pressure. These include aging, exercise, physical or emotional stress, pain, medications, and the volume of blood in circulation. For example, loss of blood will lead to abnormally low blood pressure, or hypotension. Hypotension can be life-threatening if it is not corrected.

Blood pressure is taken using a stethoscope and a blood pressure cuff, or sphygmomanometer (Fig. 11-15). Inside the cuff is an inflatable balloon that expands when air is pumped into the cuff. Two pieces of tubing are connected to the cuff. One leads to a rubber bulb that pumps air into the cuff. A pressure control button lets you control the release of air from the cuff. The other piece of tubing is connected to a pressure gauge with numbers. The gauge is either a mercury column or a round dial.

There may be an electronic sphygmomanometer available (Fig. 11-16). The systolic and diastolic pressure readings and pulse are displayed digitally. Some units automatically inflate and deflate. You do not need a stethoscope with an electronic sphygmomanometer.

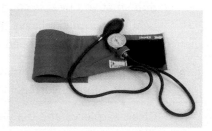

Fig. 11-15. A sphygmomanometer

When taking blood pressure, the first clear sound you will hear is the systolic pressure (top number). When the sound changes to a soft muf-

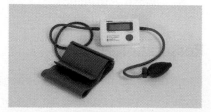

Fig. 11-16. An electronic sphygmomanometer.

fled thump or disappears, this is the diastolic pressure (bottom number). Blood pressure is recorded in a fraction. The systolic reading is on top and the diastolic reading is on the bottom (for example: 120/80).

Never measure blood pressure on an arm that has an IV, a dialysis shunt, or any medical equipment. Avoid a side that has a cast, recent trauma, or breast surgery (mastectomy).

There are two methods for taking blood pressure; they are the one-step method and the two-step method. In the two-step method, you will get an estimate of the systolic blood pressure before you start. After getting an estimated systolic reading, you will deflate the cuff and begin again. With the one-step method, you do not get an estimated systolic reading before getting the blood pressure reading. As the two-step method is generally considered safer, that is the method we will describe in this book.

Taking and recording blood pressure (two-step method)

Equipment: sphygmomanometer (blood pressure cuff), stethoscope, alcohol wipes, pen and paper

1 Wash hands.

2 Discuss what you will do.

3 Provide privacy.

4 Position your loved one's arm with palm up. The arm should be level with the heart. A false low reading is possible if the arm is above heart level.

5 With the valve open, squeeze the cuff to make sure it is completely deflated.

6 Place blood pressure cuff snugly on her upper arm, with the center of the cuff placed over the brachial artery (1-1½ inches above the elbow toward inside of elbow) (Fig. 11-17).

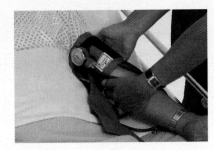

Fig. 11-17.

The cuff must be the proper size and put on arm correctly so the amount of pressure on the artery is correct. If this is not done, the reading will be falsely high or low.

7 Locate the radial (wrist) pulse with your fingertips.

8 Close the valve (clockwise) until it stops. Inflate the cuff while watching the gauge.

9 Stop inflating when you can no longer feel the radial pulse. Note the reading. The number is an estimate of the systolic pressure. This estimate helps you not to inflate the cuff too high later in this procedure. Inflating the cuff too high is painful and may damage small blood vessels.

10 Open the valve to deflate the cuff completely. An inflated cuff left on the arm can cause numbness and tingling.

11 Write down the estimated systolic reading.

12 Before using a stethoscope, wipe the diaphragm and earpieces with alcohol wipes.

13 Locate the brachial pulse with your fingertips.

14 Place the earpieces of the stethoscope in your ears.

15 Place diaphragm of stethoscope over the brachial artery.

16 Close the valve (clockwise) until it stops (Fig. 11-18). Do not tighten it. Tight valves are too hard to release.

17	Inflate cuff to 30 mm Hg above your estimated systolic pressure.
18	Open the valve slightly with thumb and index finger. Deflate cuff slowly. Releasing the valve slowly allows you to hear beats accurately.
19	Watch gauge and listen for sound of pulse.
20	Remember the reading at which the first clear pulse sound is heard. This is the systolic pressure.
21	Continue listening for a change or muffling of pulse sound. The point of a change or the point the sound disappears is the diastolic pressure. Remember this reading.
22	Open the valve to deflate cuff completely. Remove cuff.
23	Record both systolic and diastolic pressures. Write the numbers like a fraction, with the systolic reading on top and the diastolic reading on the bottom (for example, 120/80). Note which arm was used. Write "RA" for right arm and "LA" for left arm.
24	Wipe diaphragm and earpieces of stethoscope with alcohol. Store equipment.
25	Wash your hands.

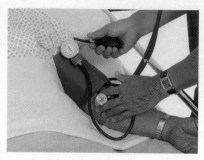

Fig. 11-18.

Pain

It is important to observe your loved one for pain. Pain is called the "fifth vital sign" because it is so important to monitor.

Pain is uncomfortable. It is also a personal experience that is different for each person; what one person thinks is painful is not for another. Treat your loved one's complaints of pain seriously and take action to help her. If your loved one complains of pain, ask these questions and report the information to her physician:

- Where is the pain?

- When did the pain start?

- Is the pain mild, moderate, or severe? To help find out, ask her to rate the pain on a scale of 1 to 10 with 10 as the worst pain imaginable.

- Ask her to describe the pain. Make notes if you need to. Use her words when reporting to the physician.

- Ask her what she was doing before the pain started.

Remember that some people do not feel comfortable saying that they are in pain. Watch for body language or other messages that your loved one may be in pain. Signs and symptoms of pain include:

- increased pulse, respirations, and/or blood pressure

- sweating

- nausea

- vomiting

- tightening the jaw

- squeezing the eyes shut

- holding a body part tightly

- frowning (Fig. 11-19)

- grinding teeth

- increased restlessness

- agitation

- change in behavior

- crying

- sighing

- groaning

- breathing heavily

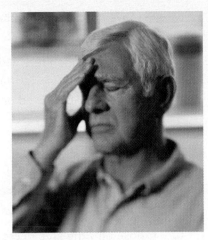

Fig. 11-19.

Measures to reduce pain include:

- Report complaints of pain or unrelieved pain to the physician promptly.

- Gently position the body in good alignment. Use pillows for support. Help with changes of position if your loved one wishes.

- Give back rubs.

- Offer warm baths or showers.

- Help your loved one to the bathroom or commode or offer the bedpan or urinal.

- Encourage slow, deep breaths if your loved one has trouble breathing.

- Provide a calm and quiet environment. Try using music as a distraction.

- Be patient, caring, gentle and sympathetic.

Catheter Care

A catheter is a tube used to drain urine from the bladder. A straight catheter does not remain inside the person; it is removed immediately after the urine is drained. An indwelling catheter remains inside the bladder for a period of time (11-20). The urine drains into a bag. An external, or condom, catheter has an attachment on the end that fits onto the penis (Fig. 11-21). The attachment is fastened with a Velcro strap or self-adhesive strip. The external catheter is changed daily.

GUIDELINES
Catheters

The drainage bag must always be kept lower than the hips or bladder. Urine must never flow from the bag or tubing back into the bladder as this can cause infection.

Tubing should be kept as straight as possible and should not be kinked. Kinks,

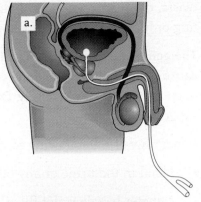

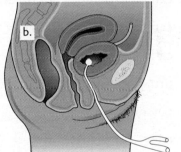

Fig. 11-20. a. An indwelling catheter (male). b. An indwelling catheter (female).

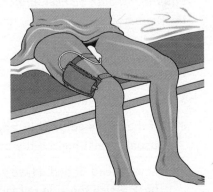

Fig. 11-21. An external or condom catheter (male).

twists, or pressure on the tubing (such as from the person sitting or lying on the tubing) can prevent urine from draining.

The genital area must be kept clean to prevent infection. Because the catheter goes all the way into the bladder, germs can enter the bladder more easily. Daily care of the genital area is especially important.

Report any of the following to your loved one's physician:

- blood in the urine or any other unusual appearance

- catheter bag does not fill after several hours

- catheter bag fills suddenly

- catheter is not in place

- urine leaks from the catheter

- person reports pain

- odor

Providing catheter care

Equipment: bath blanket, protective pad, bath basin, soap, bath thermometer, 2-4 washcloths, towel, gloves

1	Wash hands.
2	Discuss what you will do.
3	Provide privacy.
4	If the bed is adjustable, adjust it to a safe working level, usually waist high. If the bed is movable, lock bed wheels.
5	Lower head of bed. Have your loved one lie flat on her back. Raise the side rail farthest from you, if there are side rails.
6	Remove or fold back top bedding, keeping your loved one covered with bath blanket.
7	Test water temperature with thermometer or on your wrist and ensure it is safe. Water temperature should be 105° to 110° F. Have your loved one check water temperature. Adjust if necessary.
8	Put on gloves.
9	Place clean protective pad under her buttocks. Ask her to flex her knees and raise the buttocks off the bed by pushing against the mattress with her feet.
10	Expose only the area necessary to clean the catheter.
11	Place towel or pad under catheter tubing before washing.
12	Apply soap to wet washcloth.
13	Hold catheter near meatus to avoid tugging the catheter.
14	Clean at least four inches of catheter nearest meatus. Move in only one direction, away from meatus (Fig. 11-22). Use a clean area of the cloth for each stroke. 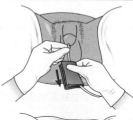
15	Dip a clean washcloth in the water. Rinse at least four inches of catheter nearest meatus. Move in only one direction, away from meatus. Use a clean area of the cloth for each stroke. 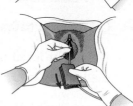

Fig. 11-22.

16	Empty the water into the toilet. Dispose of soiled linen.
17	Empty, rinse, and wipe basin and store.
18	Remove and dispose of gloves.

19   Return bed to proper level if adjusted.

20   Wash your hands.

21   Help your loved one dress and arrange the covers. Make sure the tubing is free from kinks and twists.

Emptying the catheter drainage bag

Equipment: graduate (measuring container), alcohol wipes, paper towels, disposable gloves

1   Wash your hands.

2   Discuss what you will do.

3   Provide privacy.

4   Put on gloves.

5   Place paper towel on the floor under the drainage bag. Place measuring container on the paper towel.

6   Open the drain or spout on the bag so that urine flows out of the bag into the measuring container (Fig. 11-23).

7   When urine has drained, close spout. Using alcohol wipe, clean the drain spout. Replace the drain in its holder on the bag.

8   Mentally note the amount and the appearance of the urine. Empty into toilet.

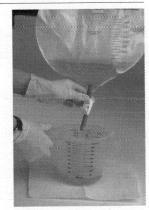

Fig. 11-23.

9   Clean and store measuring container.

10   Remove gloves.

11   Wash your hands.

12   Document the amount of urine.

Gastric Tubes

When a person is completely unable to swallow, she may be fed through a tube A nasogastric tube is inserted into the nose and goes to the stomach. A tube can also be placed through the skin directly into the stomach. This is called a PEG (Percutaneous Endoscopic Gastrostomy) tube. The opening in the stomach and abdomen is called a gastrostomy (Fig. 11-24). Tube feedings are used when a person cannot swallow but can digest food. Conditions that may prevent a person from swallowing include coma, cancer, stroke, refusal to eat, extreme weakness, or a need for increased calories.

If a person's digestive system does not function properly, hyperalimentation or total parenteral nutrition (TPN) may be needed. With TPN, a person receives nutrients directly into the bloodstream. It bypasses the digestive system.

GUIDELINES
Tube Feedings

Tubing cannot be kinked. This means it cannot be curled, twisted, or bent. Check often for kinking, especially when your loved one turns in bed or walks.

Make sure you know where tubing is when turning your

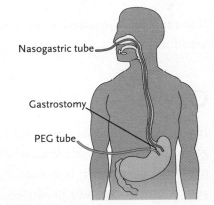

Nasogastric tube

Gastrostomy

PEG tube

Fig. 11-24.

loved one. Check to make sure that he is not on top of the tubing.

The tube is only inserted and removed by a doctor or nurse. If it comes out, report it immediately.

A doctor will prescribe the type and amount of feeding. The feedings will be in a liquid form.

During the feeding, your loved one should remain in a sitting position with the head of the bed elevated about 45 degrees.

Your loved one may have a doctor's order for "nothing by mouth," or "NPO." Be aware of this and do not give beverages if this is the case.

If your loved one must remain in bed for long periods during feedings, provide good skin care to prevent pressure sores on the hips and sacral area.

Provide frequent mouth care.

If the tubing is inserted through the abdomen, watch the site for signs of infection, including redness or drainage around the opening.

If the tubing is inserted into the nose, provide care to the nasal area for soreness and dryness.

Oxygen

If your loved one has breathing problems, he may require oxygen more concentrated than what is in the air. A doctor will prescribe oxygen if it is needed. Oxygen may be delivered to your home in tanks or produced by an oxygen concentrator. By standard convention, all oxygen tanks are green. Each oxygen tank or cylinder has a valve on top that is used to turn the oxygen on and off. There are two gauges attached to the valve; one gauge indicates how much oxygen remains in the tank and the other monitors the flow of oxygen. An oxygen concentrator changes the air in the room into air with more oxygen. The agency that supplies the oxygen will service the equipment and will provide training in its use.

Your loved one may receive oxygen through a nasal cannula (Fig. 11-25). A nasal cannula is a piece of plastic tubing that fits around the face and is secured by a strap that goes over the ears and around the back of the head. The face piece has two short prongs made of tubing. These prongs fit inside the nose and oxygen is delivered through them. A respiratory therapist fits the cannula. The length of the prongs (usually no more than half an inch) is adjusted for the person's comfort. A person can talk and eat while wearing the cannula.

A person who does not need concentrated oxygen all the time may use a face mask when he needs oxygen. The face mask fits over the nose and mouth and is secured by a strap that goes over the ears and around the back of the head. It is difficult for a person to talk when wearing an oxygen face mask. The mask must be removed for eating and drinking.

Oxygen can be irritating to the nose and mouth. The

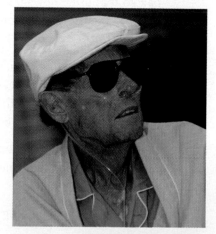

Fig. 11-25. Some people receive oxygen through a nasal cannula.

strap of a nasal cannula or face mask can also cause irritation around the ears. Wash and dry the skin carefully and provide frequent mouth care. Offer plenty of fluids. Report any irritation you observe to your loved one's physician.

Oxygen is a highly combustible gas. That means it can very easily explode or catch fire. Oxygen use requires special safety precautions.

GUIDELINES
Safety around Oxygen

Store oxygen cylinders in an upright, secure position. Do not store them in hallways or other heavy traffic areas where they may cause a fall or be knocked over.

Do not store oxygen at temperatures above 125° F. Make sure the cylinders are not covered with linens or clothing as this could raise the temperature and make the flow meter difficult to read.

Remove all fire hazards from the room or area. Fire hazards include electrical appliances, cigarettes, matches, and fluids that may catch fire easily. Examples of such fluids include alcohol and nail polish remover.

Talk to the doctor about any fire hazards that your loved one does not want removed.

Post "No Smoking" and "Oxygen in Use" signs. Never allow smoking in a room or area where oxygen is used or stored.

Never allow candles, lit matches, or other open flames around oxygen.

Learn how to turn oxygen off in case of fire. Never adjust the oxygen level.

Talk to the doctor if the nasal cannula or face mask causes irritation. Check behind the ears for irritation from tubing.

IVs

IV stands for intravenous, or into a vein. Someone with an IV is receiving medication, nutrition, or fluids through a vein. When a doctor prescribes an IV, a nurse inserts a needle into a vein, allowing direct access to the bloodstream. Medication, nutrition, or fluids either drip from a bag suspended on a pole or are pumped by a portable pump through a tube and into the vein (Fig. 11-26). If your loved one has certain chronic conditions he may have a permanent opening for an IV that has been surgically created to allow easy access for IV fluids.

Report the following about IVs to the physician:

- The needle falls out or is removed.

- The dressing around the IV site is loose or not intact.

- Blood is in the tubing or around the site of the IV.

- The site is swollen or discolored.

- Your loved one complains of pain.

- The bag is broken or the level of fluid does not seem to decrease.

- The IV fluid is not dripping.

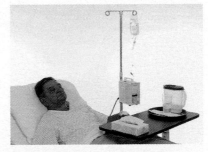

Fig. 11-26. Fluids, nutrition and medications can be delivered directly into the bloodstream through an IV.

Basic Healthcare Skills
11

- The IV fluid is nearly gone.

- The pump beeps, indicating a problem.

Collecting Specimens

You may be asked to collect a specimen, or sample, from your loved one. Different types of specimens are used for different tests. You may be asked to collect these different types of specimens:

- Sputum

- Urine (routine, clean catch/mid-stream or 24-hour)

- Stool (feces)

A "hat" is a container that is placed under the toilet seat to collect specimens from a person who uses the toilet (Fig. 11-27).

Sputum specimens are collected to check for respiratory problems. Sputum is mucus coughed up from the lungs. Early morning is the best time to collect sputum.

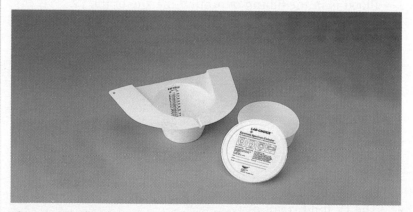

Fig. 11-27. A "hat" is used to collect specimens from a person who uses the toilet.

Collecting a sputum specimen

Equipment: specimen container with cover (labeled with your loved one's name, address, date and time), tissues, plastic bag, gloves, mask

1	Wash your hands.
2	Discuss what you will do.
3	Provide privacy.
4	Put on mask and gloves. If your loved one has known or suspected tuberculosis or another infectious disease, you should wear a mask when collecting a sputum specimen. Coughing is one way TB germs can enter the air.
5	Ask your loved one to cough deeply, so that sputum comes up from the lungs. To prevent the spread of infectious material, give him tissues to cover his mouth while coughing. Ask him to spit the sputum into the specimen container.
6	When you have obtained a good sample (about one tablespoon of sputum), cover the container tightly. Wipe any sputum off the outside of the container with tissues. Discard the tissues. Put the specimen container in the plastic bag and seal.
7	Remove gloves and mask.
8	Wash your hands.

Your loved one may be able to collect his own urine or stool specimen, or he may need your help. Be sure to explain exactly how the specimen must be collected. If specimens are not collected properly, the process may need to done over again.

Collecting a routine urine specimen

Equipment: *urine specimen container and lid, label, gloves, bedpan or urinal (if your loved one cannot use the bathroom), "hat" for toilet (if your loved one can get to the bathroom), 2 plastic bags, washcloth, towel, paper towel, supplies for perineal care, personal protective equipment (PPE) (if needed)*

1   Wash your hands.

2   Discuss what you will do.

3   Provide privacy.

4   Put on gloves.

5   Assist your loved one to the bathroom or commode, or offer the bedpan or urinal.

6   Have your loved one void into the "hat," urinal, or bedpan. Ask her not to put toilet paper in with the sample. Provide a plastic bag to discard toilet paper separately.

7   After urination, assist as necessary with perineal care. Help her wash her hands at the sink or using the washcloth and towel. Make her comfortable.

8   Take the bedpan, urinal, or "hat" to the bathroom.

9   Pour urine from the bedpan, urinal, or "hat" into the specimen container. Specimen container should be at least half full.

10 Cover the urine container with its lid. Wipe off the outside with a paper towel.

11 Place the container in a plastic bag.

12 If using a bedpan or urinal, discard extra urine. Rinse, clean, and store equipment.

13 Remove and dispose of gloves.

14 Wash your hands. Help your loved one wash his hands at the sink or using the washcloth and towel.

15 Complete the label for the container with your loved one's name, address, the date, and time.

16 Note the amount and characteristics of urine.

Collecting a clean catch (mid-stream) urine specimen

Equipment: *specimen kit with container, label, cleansing solution, gauze or towelettes, gloves, bedpan or urinal (if your loved one cannot use the bathroom), plastic bag, washcloth, paper towel, towel, supplies for perineal care, personal protective equipment (PPE) (if needed)*

1   Wash hands.

2   Discuss what you will do.

3   Provide privacy.

4   Put on gloves.

5   Open the specimen kit. Do not touch the inside of the container or the inside of the lid.

6   Using the towelettes or gauze and cleansing solution, clean the area around the urethra. **For a woman**, separate the labia and wipe from front to back along one side. Discard towelette/gauze. With a new towelette or gauze, wipe from front to back along the other labia. Using a new towelette or gauze, wipe down the middle.

For a man, clean the head of the penis using circular motions with the towelettes or gauze. Clean thoroughly, changing towelettes/gauze after each circular motion and discarding after use. If the man is uncircumcised, pull back the foreskin of the penis before cleaning and hold it back during urination. Make sure it is pulled back down after collecting the specimen. Improper cleaning can infect the urinary tract and contaminate the sample.

7	Ask your loved one to urinate into the bedpan, urinal, or toilet and to stop before urination is complete.
8	Place the container under the urine stream and have him start urinating again. Fill the container at least half full. Have him finish urinating in bedpan, urinal, or toilet.
9	Cover the urine container with its lid. Wipe off the outside with a paper towel.
10	Place the container in a plastic bag for safe transport.
11	If using a bedpan or urinal, discard extra urine. Rinse, clean and store equipment.
12	Remove and dispose of gloves. Wash your hands. Help your loved one wash his hands at the sink or using the washcloth and towel.
13	Complete the label for the container with your loved one's name, address, the date, and time.
14	Wash your hands.

When collecting a 24-hour urine specimen, you may not be present during all 24 hours of the test. It is important to explain the collection fully to your loved one and anyone else who may be in the home to assist. All urine must be collected and stored properly. If any is accidentally thrown away or improperly stored, the collection will have to be done over again.

Collecting a 24-hour urine specimen

Equipment: 24-hour specimen container, label, bedpan or urinal (if your loved one is confined to bed), "hat" for toilet (if she can get to the bathroom), bucket of ice if the urine must be kept cold (a clearly marked container can also be put in the refrigerator), gloves, plastic bag, washcloth or towel, supplies for perineal care, personal protective equipment (PPE) (if needed)

1	Wash your hands.
2	Explain what you will do.
3	Provide privacy.
4	When beginning the collection, have your loved one completely empty her bladder. Discard the urine and note the exact time of this voiding. The collection will run until the same time the next day.
5	Label the container with your loved one's name, address, dates and times the collection period began and ended (Fig. 11-28).

Client:
Josie Montoya

Address:
8529 Indian School
Albuquerque, NM 87112

Date Time
Begin Collection: 7/6/05 7:00am
End Collection: 7/7/05 7:00am

| 6 | Put on gloves each time your loved one voids. |

Fig. 11-28.

| 7 | Pour urine from bedpan, urinal, or "hat" into the container. Container may be stored on ice or in the refrigerator if clearly marked. |
| 8 | After each voiding, help as necessary with perineal care. Offer handwashing supplies after each voiding. |

9   Be sure everyone understands that all urine is to be saved, even if you are gone when it is voided. Show them how to pour the urine into the container and remind them to store the container in the bucket of ice or in the refrigerator if ordered.

10   Clean equipment after each voiding.

11   After the last void of the 24-hour period, add the urine to the specimen container. Place container in the plastic bag.

12   Remove gloves.

13   Wash your hands.

14   Document the time of the last void before the 24-hour collection period began, and the last void of the 24-hour collection period.

When collecting a stool specimen, ask your loved one to let you know when she can have a bowel movement. Be ready to collect the specimen. Do not get urine or tissue in the sample. Urine and paper can ruin the sample.

Collecting a stool specimen

Equipment: *specimen container and lid with label, 2 tongue blades, 2 pair gloves, bedpan (if your loved one cannot use the bathroom or commode), "hat" (if using toilet or commode), 2 plastic bags, toilet tissue, washcloth or towel, supplies for perineal care, personal protective equipment (PPE) (if needed)*

1   Wash your hands.

2   Discuss what you will do.

3   Provide privacy.

4   Put on gloves.

5   When your loved one is ready to move her bowels, ask her to try not to urinate at the same time and not to put toilet paper in with the sample. Provide a plastic bag to discard toilet paper separately. Urine and paper contaminate the sample.

6   Fit "hat" to toilet or commode, or provide the bedpan. Leave the room and ask her to signal when she is finished with the bowel movement. Make sure she has a way to call you and be ready to return.

7   After the bowel movement, assist as necessary with perineal care. Help your loved one wash her hands at the sink or using the washcloth and towel. Make her comfortable. Remove gloves.

8   Wash your hands again.

9   Put on clean gloves.

10   Using the two tongue blades, take about two tablespoons of stool and put it in the container. Cover it tightly.

11   Wrap the tongue blades in toilet paper and throw them away. Empty the bedpan or container into the toilet. Clean and store the equipment.

12   Complete the label for the container with your loved one's name, address, the date, and time. Bag the specimen.

13   Remove and dispose of gloves.

14   Wash your hands.

Non-Sterile Dressings

Sterile dressings are those that cover open or draining wounds.

These dressings are usually changed by a nurse. Non-sterile dressings are applied to dry wounds that have less chance of infection.

Changing a dry dressing using non-sterile technique

Equipment: package of square gauze dressings, adhesive tape, scissors, 2 pair of gloves

1   Wash your hands.

2   Discuss what you will be doing.

3   Provide privacy.

4   Cut pieces of tape long enough to secure the dressing. Hang tape on the edge of a table within reach. Open the four-inch square gauze package without touching the gauze. Place the opened package on a flat surface.

5   Put on gloves.

6   Remove soiled dressing by gently peeling the tape toward the wound. Lift the dressing off the wound. Do not drag it over the wound. Observe dressing for any odor. Notice the color of the wound. Dispose of used dressing in proper container. Remove and dispose of gloves.

7   Put on new gloves. Touching only the outer edges of new four-inch gauze, remove it from package. Apply it to wound. Tape gauze in place. Secure it firmly (Fig. 11-29). Keep gauze as clean as possible.

Fig. 11-29.

8   Remove and dispose of gloves properly.

9   Wash your hands.

10   Note any observations.

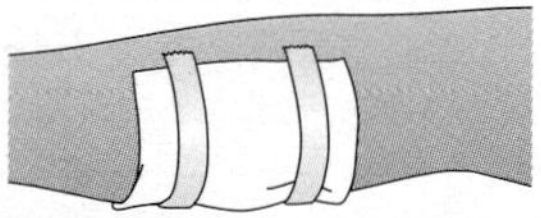

Warm and Cold Applications

Applying heat or cold to injured areas can have several beneficial effects. Heat relieves pain and muscular tension. It decreases swelling, elevates the temperature in the tissues, and increases blood flow. Increased blood flow brings more oxygen and nutrients to the tissues for healing.

Cold can help stop bleeding. It prevents swelling and reduces pain. Cold helps bring down high fevers.

Warm and cold applications may be dry or moist. Moisture strengthens the effect of heat and cold. This means that moist applications are more likely to cause injury. Be careful when using these applications. Know how long the application should be performed. Use the correct temperature as specified by the doctor. Check on the application as directed.

Types of dry applications are:

- Aquamatic K-pad ® (warm or cold) (Fig. 11-30).

- Electric heating pad (warm)

- Disposable warm pack (warm)

- Ice bag (cold)

- Disposable cold pack (cold)

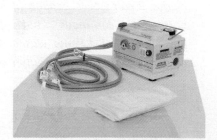

Fig. 11-30.

Types of moist applications are:

- Compresses (warm or cold)

- Soaks (warm or cold)

- Tub baths (warm)

- Sitz baths (warm)

- Ice packs (cold)

Report to the doctor if any of the following occur with warm or cold applications:

- excessive redness

- pain

- blisters

- numbness

If you observe these signs, the application may be causing tissue damage.

Applying warm compresses

Equipment: *washcloth or compress, plastic wrap, towel, basin, bath thermometer*

1   Wash your hands.

2   Explain what you will do.

3   Provide privacy as needed.

4   Fill basin one-half to two-thirds full with hot water. Check temperature with thermometer (should be between 105°F and 110° F), or against the inside of your wrist. Have your loved once check water temperature and adjust if necessary.

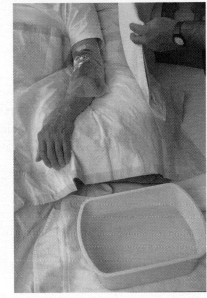

Fig. 11-31.

5   Soak the washcloth in the water and wring it out. Immediately apply it to the area needing a warm compress. Note the time. Quickly cover the washcloth with plastic wrap and the towel to keep it warm (Fig. 11-31).

6   Check the area every five minutes. Remove the compress if the area is red or numb or if your loved one complains of pain or discomfort. Change the compress if cooling occurs. Remove the compress after 20 minutes.

7   Commercial warm compresses are also available. If using these, follow the package directions and any instructions from the doctor.

8   Discard water in the toilet. Clean and store basin and other supplies. Put laundry in hamper. Discard plastic wrap.

9   Wash your hands.

10   Note any observations.

Administering warm soaks

Equipment: towel, basin, bath thermometer, bath blanket

1   Wash your hands.

2   Discuss what you will do.

3   Provide privacy.

4   Fill the basin or tub half full of warm water. Check temperature with thermometer (should be between 105°F and 110°F), or against the inside of your wrist. Have your loved once check water temperature and adjust if necessary.

5   Immerse the body part in the basin, or help your loved one into the tub. Pad the edge of the basin with a towel if needed (Fig. 11-32). Use a bath blanket to cover the rest of your loved one's body if needed for extra warmth.

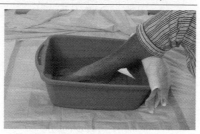

Fig. 11-32.

6   Check water temperature every five minutes and add hot water as needed to maintain the temperature. Never add water hotter than 110° F. To prevent burns, be sure your loved one does not add water herself. Observe the area for redness and discontinue the soak if she complains of pain or discomfort.

7   Soak for 15-20 minutes, or as ordered by the doctor.

8   Remove basin and use the towel to dry her off.

9   Discard water. Clean and store basin and other supplies. Put laundry in hamper.

10 Wash your hands.

11 Note any observations, especially observations about the skin.

Using a hot water bottle

Equipment: hot water bottle, cloth cover or towel, bath thermometer

1   Wash your hands.

2   Discuss what you will do.

3   Provide privacy as needed.

4   Fill the bottle half full with warm water (105° F–115° F, or 98° F–110° F for older adults).

5   Press out excess air and seal the bottle.

6   Dry the bottle and check for leaks. Cover with a cloth cover or towel.

7   Apply the bottle to the area ordered. Check skin every five minutes for redness or pain. If redness or pain are present, add cold water to the bottle to reduce the temperature.

8   Remove the bottle after 20 minutes or as ordered by the doctor.

9   Empty the hot water bottle. Wash and store supplies.

10 Wash your hands.

11 Note any observations, especially observations about the skin.

A sitz bath is a warm soak of the perineal area. Sitz baths clean perineal wounds and reduce inflammation and pain. Circulation is increased and voiding may be stimulated by a sitz bath. People with perineal swelling (such as hemorrhoids) may be ordered to take sitz baths. Because the sitz bath causes increased blood flow to the pelvic area, blood flow to other parts of the body decreases. A person may feel weak, faint, or dizzy after a sitz bath. Always wear gloves when helping with a sitz bath.

Assisting with a sitz bath

Equipment: disposable sitz bath, bath thermometer, towels, gloves

A disposable sitz bath fits on the toilet seat and is attached to a rubber bag containing warm water (Fig. 11-33).

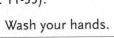

Fig. 11-33.

1   Wash your hands.

2   Discuss what you will do.

3   Provide privacy.

4   Put on gloves.

5   Fill the sitz bath two-thirds full with hot water. Place the disposable sitz bath on the toilet seat. If the sitz bath is prescribed for cleaning the perineal area, the temperature should be 100° F–104° F. For a sitz bath given for pain and to stimulate circulation, the water temperature should be 105°F–110° F. Check the water temperature using the bath thermometer.

6   Help your loved one undress and be seated on the sitz bath. A valve on the tubing connected to the bag allows her or you to replenish the water in the sitz bath with hot water.

7   Leave the room, but check on her every five minutes to make sure she is not dizzy or weak. Stay with her if she seems unsteady.

8   Assist her out of the sitz bath in 20 minutes. Provide towels and help with dressing if needed.

9   Clean and store supplies.

10 Remove your gloves.

11 Wash your hands.

12 Note any observations.

Applying ice packs

Equipment: ice pack or sealable plastic bag and crushed ice, towel to cover pack or bag

1   Wash your hands.

2   Explain what you will do.

3   Provide privacy as needed.

4   Fill the plastic bag one-half to two-thirds full with crushed ice. Remove excess air. Cover bag or ice pack with towel (Fig. 11-34).

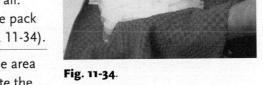

Fig. 11-34.

5   Apply bag to the area as ordered. Note the time. Use another towel to cover the bag if it is too cold.

6   Check the area after ten minutes for blisters or pale, white, or gray skin. Stop treatment if your loved one complains of numbness or pain.

7   Remove ice after 20 minutes or as ordered.

8   Return ice bag or pack to freezer.

9 Wash your hands.

10 Note any observations, especially observations about the skin.

Applying cold compresses

Equipment: basin filled with water and ice, two washcloths, plastic or rubber sheet, towels

1 Wash your hands.

2 Discuss what you will do.

3 Provide privacy as needed.

4 Position your loved one on the plastic sheet. Rinse washcloth in basin and wring it out. Cover the area to be treated with a cloth sheet or towel and apply a cold washcloth

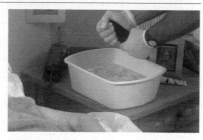

Fig. 11-35.

to the area as directed (Fig. 11-35). Change washcloths often to keep the area cold.

5 Check the area after five minutes for blisters or pale, white, or gray skin. Stop treatment if your loved one complains of numbness or pain.

6 Remove compresses after 20 minutes or as ordered. Provide towels as needed to dry the area.

7 Clean and store basin.

8 Wash your hands.

9 Note any observations, especially any observations about the skin.

Anti-Embolic Hose

For some cases of poor circulation to legs and feet, elastic stockings are ordered. These special stockings help prevent swelling and embolisms. An embolism is a blood clot. Blood clots can be very serious. These stockings, called anti-embolic hose, or TED hose, promote circulation. Follow the manufacturer's instructions and illustrations on how to put on stockings.

Applying anti-embolic hose

Equipment: anti-embolic hose

1 Wash your hands.

2 Discuss what you will do.

3 Provide privacy as needed.

4 With your loved one lying down, remove his socks, shoes, or slippers, and expose one leg.

5 Turn stocking inside-out at least to heel area (Fig. 11-36).

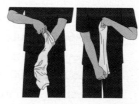

Fig. 11-36.

6 Gently place the foot of the stocking over toes, foot, and heel (Fig. 11-37). Make sure the heel is in the right place.

7 Gently pull top of stocking over foot, heel, and leg (Fig. 11-38).

8 Make sure that there are no twists or wrinkles in the stocking after it is applied. It must fit smoothly. If you have trouble put-

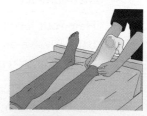

Fig. 11-37.

ting the stocking on, try applying powder to your loved one's leg before pulling stocking up.

9	Repeat for the other leg.
10	Wash your hands.
11	Note any observations.

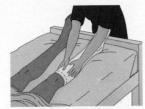

Fig. 11-38.

Range of Motion Exercises

Exercise helps people regain strength and mobility. It prevents disabilities from developing. People who are in bed for long periods of time are more likely to develop contractures. A contracture is the permanent and often very painful stiffening of a joint and muscle. They are generally caused by immobility. Contractures can result in the loss of ability.

Range of motion (ROM) exercises are exercises that put a particular joint through its full arc of motion. The purpose of range of motion exercises is to decrease or prevent contractures, improve strength, and increase circulation. Passive range of motion (PROM) exercises are used when a person is not able to move on his own. When assisting with PROM exercises, support your loved one's joints and move them through the range of motion. Active range of motion (AROM) exercises are performed by the person on his own. Your role in AROM exercises is to encourage your loved one. Active assisted range of motion (AAROM) exercises are performed by your loved one with some assistance and support from you or a healthcare professional.

You will not do ROM exercises without an order from a doctor or physical therapist. You will repeat each exercise two to five times, once or twice a day. You will work on both sides of the body. During ROM exercises, begin at your loved one's head and work down the body. Exercise the upper extremities (arms) before the lower extremities (legs). Give support above and below the joint. Stop the motion if your loved one reports pain; report any complaints of pain to the doctor. These exercises are specific for each body area; they include the movements below (Fig. 11-39):

- Abduction: moving a body part away from the body

- Adduction: moving a body part toward the body

- Dorsiflexion: bending backward

- Rotation: turning a joint

- Extension: straightening a body part

- Flexion: bending a body part

- Pronation: turning downward

- Supination: turning upward

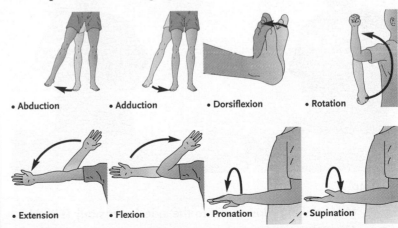

Fig. 11-39.

Assisting with passive range of motion exercises

1   Wash your hands.

2   Discuss what you will do.

3   Provide privacy as needed.

4   If bed is adjustable, adjust it to a safe level, usually waist high. If bed is movable, lock bed wheels.

5   Position your loved one supine—lying flat on his or her back—on the bed. Use good alignment.

6   **Shoulder**. Support the arm at the elbow and wrist during ROM for the shoulder. Place one hand above the elbow and the other hand around the wrist. Move the arm upward so that the upper arm is aligned with the side of the head (forward flexion) (Fig. 11-40).

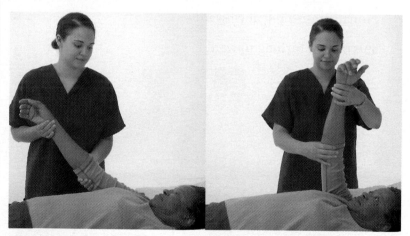

Fig. 11-40.

Move the arm downward to the side (extension) (Fig. 11-41). Return arm to side.

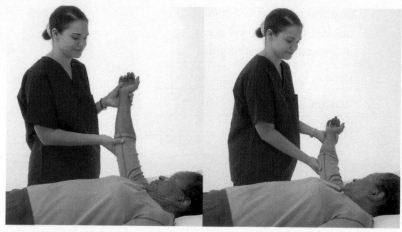

Fig. 11-41.

Bring the arm sideways away from the body to above the head (abduction) (Fig. 11-42) and back down (adduction).

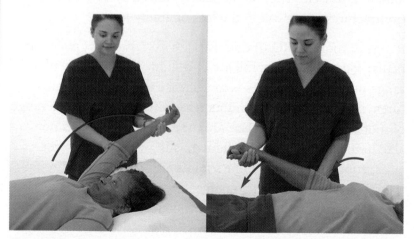

Fig. 11-42.

Bend the elbow and position it at the same level as the shoulder. Move the forearm down toward the midline of the body (internal rotation). Now move the forearm toward the head (external rotation) (Fig. 11-43).

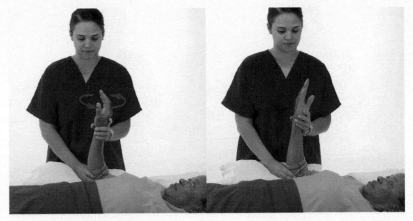

Fig. 11-45.

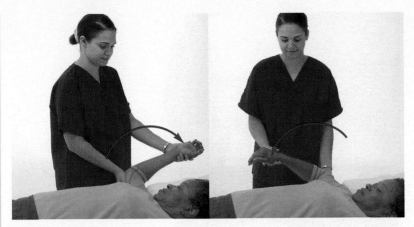

Fig. 11-43.

7   **Elbow**. Hold your loved one's wrist with one hand, the elbow with the other hand. Bend the elbow so that the hand touches the shoulder on that same side (flexion). Straighten the arm (extension) (Fig. 11-44).

8   **Wrist**. Hold the wrist with one hand and use the fingers of the other hand to help the joint through the motions. Bend the hand down (flexion); bend the hand backwards (extension) (Fig. 11-46).

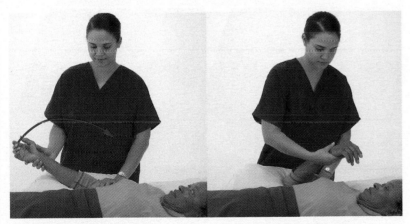

Fig. 11-44.

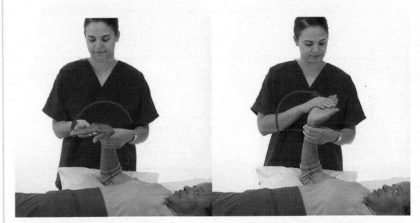

Fig. 11-46.

Exercise the forearm by moving it so the palm is facing downward (pronation) and then the palm is facing upward (supination) (Fig. 11-45).

Turn the hand in the direction of the thumb (radial flexion); turn the hand in the direction of the little finger (ulnar flexion) (Fig. 11-47).

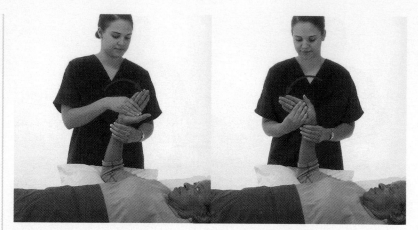

Fig. 11-47.

9   **Thumb**. Move the thumb away from the index finger (abduction). Move the thumb back next to the index finger (adduction) (Fig. 11-48).

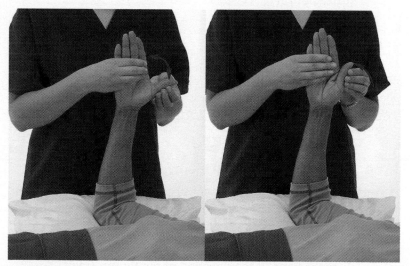

Fig. 11-48.

Touch each fingertip with the thumb (opposition) (Fig. 11-49).

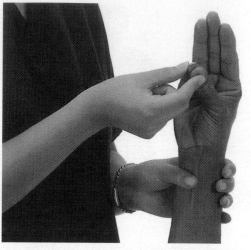

Fig. 11-49.

Bend thumb into the palm (flexion) and out to the side (extension) (Fig. 11-50).

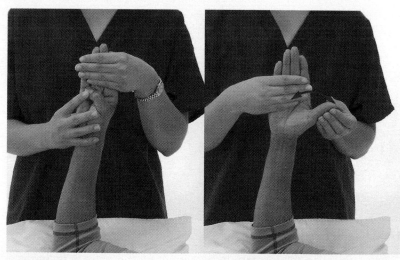

Fig. 11-50.

10   **Fingers**. Make the hand into a fist (flexion). Gently straighten out the fist (extension) (Fig. 11-51).

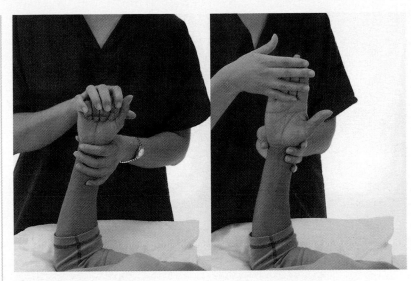

Fig. 11-51.

Spread the fingers and the thumb far apart from each other (abduction). Bring the fingers back next to each other (adduction) (Fig. 11-52).

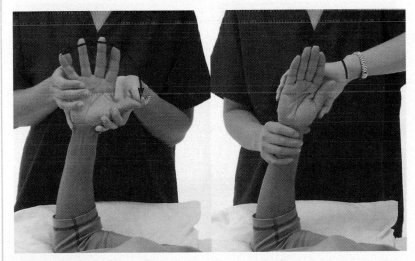

Fig. 11-52.

11 **Hip**. Support the leg by placing one hand under the knee and one under the ankle. Straighten the leg and raise it gently upward. Move the leg away from the other leg (abduction). Move the leg toward the other leg (adduction) (Fig. 11-53).

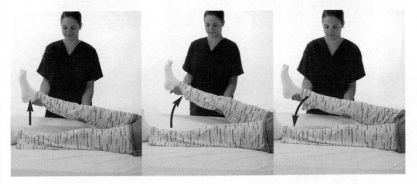

Fig. 11-53.

Gently turn the leg inward (internal rotation), then turn the leg outward (external rotation) (Fig. 11-54).

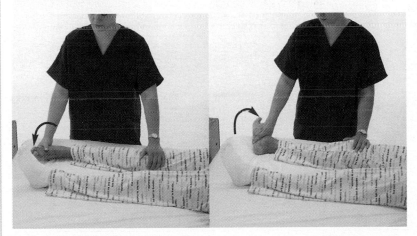

Fig. 11-54.

12 **Knees**. Bend the leg at the knee (flexion). Straighten the leg (extension) (Fig. 11-55).

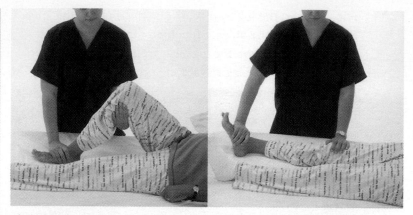

Fig. 11-55.

13 **Ankles**. Bend the foot up toward the leg (dorsiflexion). Turn the foot down away from the leg (plantar flexion) (Fig. 11-56).

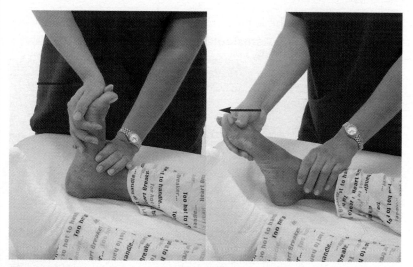

Fig. 11-56.

Turn the inside of the foot inward toward the body (supination). Bend the sole of the foot so that it faces away from the body (pronation) (Fig. 11-57).

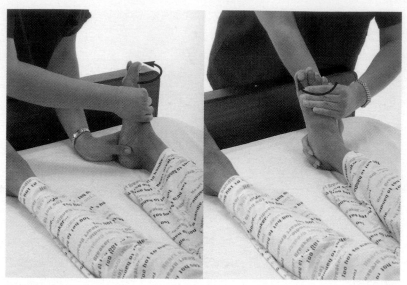

Fig. 11-57.

14 **Toes**. Curl and straighten the toes (flexion and extension) (Fig. 11-58).

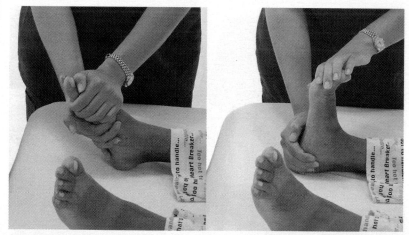

Fig. 11-58.

Gently spread the toes apart (abduction) (Fig. 11-59).

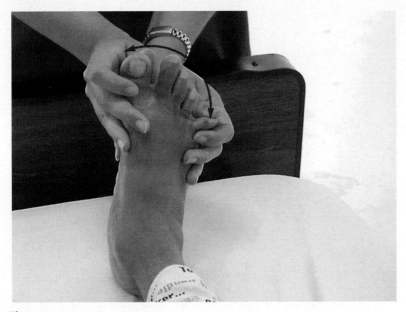

Fig. 11-59

15 Return your loved one to a comfortable resting position and cover as appropriate. If you raised an adjustable bed, lower it to its proper position.

16 Wash your hands.

17 Note any observations. Note any decrease in range of motion or any pain experienced. Notify the doctor if you find increased stiffness or physical resistance. Resistance may be a sign that a contracture is developing.

Deep Breathing Exercises

Deep breathing exercises help expand the lungs, clearing them of mucus and preventing infections (such as pneumonia). People who are paralyzed or who have had abdominal surgery are often told to do deep breathing exercises regularly to expand the lungs. Do not assist with these exercises if you have not been trained. Ask your doctor for instruction. The following procedure is intended as general instruction only.

Assisting with deep breathing exercises

Equipment: 2 pairs of gloves, tissues, waste container, small basin, oral care supplies

1 Wash your hands.

2 Discuss what you will do.

3 Provide privacy as desired.

4 Put on a mask, goggles, and gown as indicated by Standard Precautions. Use other PPE as directed by your doctor.

5 Put on gloves.

6 With your loved one sitting up if possible, have him breathe in as deeply as possible through the nose. You should see the chest and then the abdomen expand and fill with air.

7 Have him exhale through the mouth until all air is expelled.

8 Repeat this exercise five to ten times, as specified by the doctor.

9 If your loved one coughs or brings up mucus from the lungs during the exercise, offer tissues or the basin to catch the mucus.

10 Dispose of the used tissues and clean the basin.

Basic Healthcare Skills

11

11	Remove gloves, goggles, mask, and gown.
12	Wash your hands.
13	Put on fresh gloves.
14	Provide mouth care as desired, and help your loved one return to a comfortable position.
15	Remove your gloves.
16	Wash your hands again.
17	Note any observations or reactions, including pain, prolonged coughing, and color or amount of mucus.

12

Healthy Eating and Hydration

The importance of good nutrition must not be underestimated. For the human body to grow new cells, maintain normal functioning of all systems, and have energy for activities, it needs a well-balanced diet containing essential nutrients and adequate fluids.

For those who are ill or elderly, a well-balanced, nutritious diet helps maintain muscle and skin tissues and prevent pressure sores. A good diet also promotes the healing of wounds and helps a person cope with physical and emotional stress.

First Steps

Talk to your loved one and her physician and find out if she has any special concerns or conditions that could affect her appetite or her nutritional intake. Would she benefit from a diet of thickened liquids or from assistive devices for eating? Remember that one of the major goals of caregiving is to allow your loved one as much independence as possible.

Find out your loved one's food and beverage likes and dislikes. Offering food and drink that is appealing to her will help you ensure that she receives optimal nutrition and avoids dehydration.

Do not forget about yourself! While you are monitoring your loved one's nutrition, work on a healthier diet for yourself as well. Good nutrition and hydration will allow you to function more effectively as a caregiver as well as in other areas of your life.

Aging and Illness

Aging and illness can lead to emotional and physical problems that affect the intake of food. For example, people who are lonely or depressed may have little interest in food. Weaker hands and arms due to paralysis or tremors make it hard to eat. People with illnesses that affect their ability to chew and swallow may not want to eat. Special care must be taken in meal planning and preparation to ensure good nutrition.

Physical changes due to aging that may affect nutrition include the following:

- Metabolism slows. Muscles weaken and lose tone. Body movement slows. Reduced activity or exercise affects appetite.

- Loss of vision may affect the way food looks. This may decrease appetite.

- Weakened sense of smell and taste affect appetite. Medication may impair these senses (Fig. 12-1).

- Less saliva production affects chewing and swallowing.

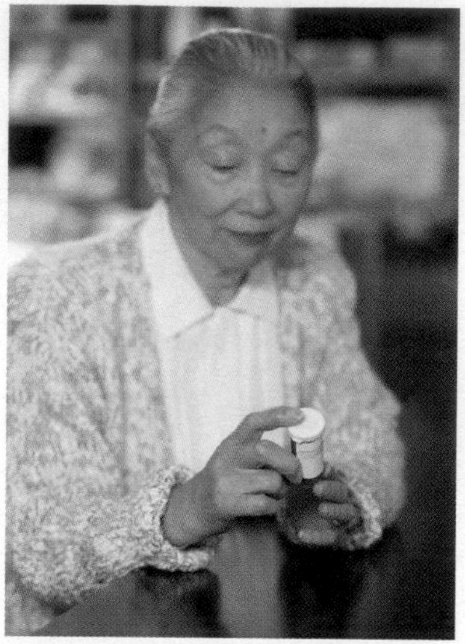

Fig. 12-1. Many elderly people are taking a variety of medications, which can affect the way food smells and tastes.

- Dentures, tooth loss, or poor dental health make chewing difficult.

- Digestion takes longer and is less efficient.

Medications or limited activity may cause constipation. Constipation may interfere with appetite; fiber, fluids, and exercise can help.

Many illnesses require restrictions in fluids, proteins, certain minerals, or calories (Fig. 12-2). In addition, people who are ill are often tired, nauseated, or in pain. This contributes to poor fluid and food intake. Conditions that make eating or swallowing difficult include:

- Stroke, or CVA, which can cause weakness and paralysis

- Nerve and muscle damage from head and neck cancer

- Multiple Sclerosis
- Parkinson's disease
- Alzheimer's disease

If your loved one has trouble swallowing, soft foods and thickened liquids should be served. A straw or special cup will help make swallowing easier. Swallowing problems cause a high risk for choking on food or drink. Inhaling food or drink into the lungs is called aspiration. Aspiration can cause pneumonia or death. Alert the doctor as soon as possible if any problems occur while your loved one is eating.

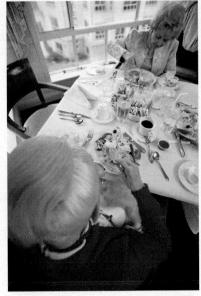

Fig. 12-2. Many illnesses require food restrictions.

Preventing Aspiration

Position your loved one properly when eating. She should sit in a straight, upright position; do not try to feed her in a reclining position.

Offer small pieces of food or small spoonfuls of pureed food.

Feed your loved one slowly.

Place food in the non-paralyzed, or unaffected, side of the mouth.

Make sure the mouth is empty before each bite of food or sip of drink.

Your loved one should stay in the upright position for about 30 minutes after eating and drinking.

Basic Nutrients

The body needs the following nutrients for growth and development:

1. **Protein**. Proteins are part of every body cell, and are essential for tissue growth and repair. Proteins are also an alternate supply of energy for the body. Sources of protein include fish, seafood, poultry, meat, eggs, milk, cheese, nuts, peas, and dried beans (Fig. 12-3). Whole grain cereals, pastas, rice, and breads contain some proteins of lower quality, which must be combined with more complete proteins. Beans and rice, or cereal and milk, are examples of complementary proteins.

2. **Carbohydrates**. Carbohydrates supply the fuel for the body's energy needs. They help the body use fat efficiently. Carbohydrates also provide fiber, which is necessary for bowel elimination. Carbohydrates can be divided into two basic types: 1) complex carbohydrates, which are found in foods such as bread, cereal, potatoes, rice, pasta, vegetables, and fruits and 2) simple

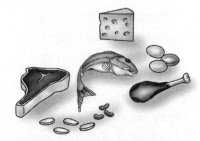

Fig. 12-3. Sources of protein.

Healthy Eating and Hydration **12**

carbohydrates, found in foods such as sugars, sweets, syrups, and jellies (Fig. 12-4). Simple carbohydrates do not have the same nutritional value as complex carbohydrates.

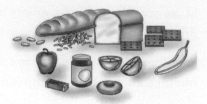

Fig. 12-4. Sources of carbohydrates.

The only value of simple carbohydrates is as energy for people who eat very little or are malnourished. For others, simple carbohydrates offer no nutritional benefit and may contribute to excess weight gain.

3. **Fats.** Fat helps the body store energy, provides the body with insulation and protects body organs. Fats add flavor to food and are important for the absorption of certain vitamins. Excess fat in the diet is stored as fat in the body. Examples of fats are butter, margarine, salad dressings, oils, and animal fats in meats, fowl, and fish (Fig. 12-5). Monounsaturated vegetable fats (including olive oil and canola oil) and polyunsaturated vegetable fats (including corn and safflower oils) are healthier fats. Saturated fats, including animal fats like butter, lard, bacon and other fatty meats, are not as healthy and should be limited.

4. **Vitamins.** Vitamins are substances the body needs to function (Fig. 12-6). The body cannot produce most vitamins; they can only be obtained from food. But they are essential to body func-

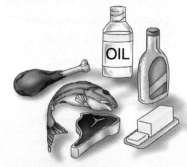

Fig. 12-5. Sources of fats.

VITAMIN	SOURCE	FUNCTION
Vitamin A	dark green and yellow vegetables, such as broccoli and turnips	assists with skin and eye development, keeps the skin healthy, helps the eyes adjust to dim light, helps the linings of the respiratory and digestive tracts resist infection
Vitamin C	fruits such as oranges, strawberries, grapefruit, cantaloupe; and vegetables such as broccoli, cabbage, brussels sprouts, and green peppers	assists with healing wounds and building bones and teeth, holds cells together, strengthens the walls of blood vessels, and helps the body absorb iron
Vitamin B2 or riboflavin	milk, milk products, lean meat, green leafy vegetables, eggs, breads, and cereals	helps cells use oxygen, which allows them to release energy from food; important for protein and carbohydrate metabolism; needed for growth, healthy eyes, skin, and mucous membranes
Vitamin B3 or niacin	lean meat, poultry, fish, peanuts and peanut butter, whole grain breads and cereals, peas, beans, and eggs	important for protein, carbohydrate and fat metabolism, appetite, and the functioning of the skin, tongue, nervous system, and digestive system; helps cells use oxygen for energy

VITAMIN	SOURCE	FUNCTION
Vitamin D	milk, butter, liver, and fish liver oils; also obtained by exposing the body to direct sunlight, which interacts with the cholesterol in the skin	responsible for the body's absorption of the minerals calcium and phosphorus and contributes to the formation of healthy bones; especially important to growing children and women who are pregnant or breastfeeding
Thiamin	lean pork, dried beans, peas, whole grain and enriched breads and cereals, and certain types of nuts	helps the body obtain energy from foods

Fig. 12-6. Source and function of essential vitamins.

tions. Vitamins A, D, E, and K are fat-soluble vitamins, meaning they are carried and stored in body fat. Vitamins B and C are water-soluble vitamins that are broken down by water in our bodies. They cannot be stored in the body, but are eliminated in urine and feces.

5. **Minerals**. Minerals help maintain cell functions (Fig. 12-7). They provide energy and regulate processes. Zinc, iron, calcium, and magnesium are some minerals. Minerals are found in many foods.

6. **Water**. Because one-half to two-thirds of our body weight is water, we need about eight glasses, or 64 ounces, of water a day. Water is the most essential nutrient for life. Without it, a person can only live for a few days. Water assists in the

MINERAL	SOURCE	FUNCTION
Iron	egg yolks, green leafy vegetables, breads, cereals, and organ meats	necessary for the red blood cells to carry oxygen, helps in the formation of enzymes
Sodium	almost all foods and table salt	important for maintaining fluid balance (helps the body retain water)
Calcium	milk and milk products such as cheese, ice cream, and yogurt; green leafy vegetables such as collards, kale, mustard, dandelion, and turnip greens; and canned fish with soft bones, such as salmon	important for the formation of teeth and bones, the clotting of blood, muscle contraction, and heart and nerve function
Potassium	fruits and vegetables, cereals, coffee, and meats	essential for nerve and heart function and muscle contraction
Phosphorus	milk, milk products, meat, fish, poultry, nuts, and eggs	needed for the formation of bones and teeth and nerve and heart function; important for the body's utilization of proteins, fats, and carbohydrates

Fig. 12-7. Source and function of essential minerals.

digestion and absorption of food as well as the elimination of waste. Through perspiration, water also helps maintain normal body temperature. Keeping enough fluid in our bodies is necessary for good health.

The USDA Food Guide Pyramid

Most foods contain several nutrients, but no one food contains all the nutrients that are necessary to maintain a healthy body. Therefore, it is important that we eat a daily diet that is well-balanced.

The U.S. Department of Agriculture (USDA) has divided the foods that we eat into six groups:

1. grains, including cereals, bread, rice, and pasta

2. fruits

3. vegetables

4. milk and milk products

5. meat, poultry, fish, eggs, dry beans, and nuts

6. fats, oils, and sweets

These six groups have been arranged into the Food Guide Pyramid (Fig. 12-8). Foods close to the bottom of the pyramid should make up most of our diet. Foods closer to the top should be eaten in smaller quantities.

Grains. Grains are found in cereal, bread, rice, and pasta. The Food Guide Pyramid recommends eating between six and eleven servings from the grain group each day. Examples of one serving include one slice of bread, one cup of dry cereal, or 1/2 cup of cooked pasta, cereal or rice. Grains are an excellent source of carbohydrates. Complex carbohydrates take longer to

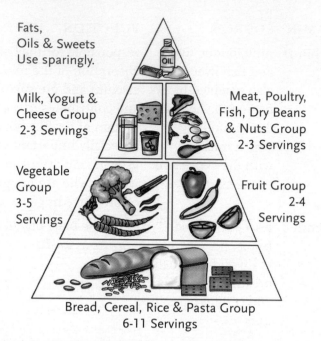

Fig. 12-8. The Food Guide Pyramid was created by the U.S. Department of Agriculture. The six food groups together make up a healthy diet.

break down and provide longer-lasting energy than simple carbohydrates. Whole grain foods, such as whole wheat breads, bran cereals, brown rice, and whole wheat pastas contain more complex carbohydrates than white breads, rice, pastas, and processed cereals. Whole grain foods also contain more vitamins, protein, and energy.

Vegetables. Vegetables are excellent sources of vitamins and fiber. Choose from green leafy vegetables such as lettuce, spinach, and kale, tomatoes, green beans, peas, corn, cabbage, cauliflower, broccoli, and other vegetables. Vegetable sources of vitamin C include brussels sprouts, green and red peppers, and broccoli. The Food Guide Pyramid recommends eating three to five servings from the vegetable group each day. One serving from this group consists of one cup of raw, leafy vegetables, 1/2 cup of cooked or chopped vegetables, or 3/4 cup of vegetable juice.

Fruits. Fruits are good sources of complex carbohydrates, vitamins, and fiber. Fruits are among the best sources of vitamin C, a nutrient we should consume each day. Good sources of vitamin C include oranges and orange juice, grapefruit and grapefruit juice, strawberries, mango, papaya, and cantaloupe. The Food Guide Pyramid recommends eating two to four servings from the fruit group each day. One serving from this group could include one medium-sized apple, orange, pear, or banana; 3/4 cup of juice; or 1/2 cup of chopped, cooked, or canned fruit.

Dairy Products. Milk and milk products, such as cheese and yogurt, are good sources of calcium, a nutrient needed for healthy bones and teeth (Fig 12-9). Milk products also contain other minerals, protein, and vitamins. Other milk products include buttermilk, evaporated milk, and cottage cheese. Whole milk, cheese, and other products made with whole milk contain a lot of saturated fat. Most adults should eat low-fat or nonfat milk and milk products. Adults should have two to three servings from the dairy group each day. One serving is one cup of milk or yogurt, 1/2 cup of cottage cheese, or 1 1/2 ounces of natural cheese.

For people who dislike milk, powdered milk can be used in cooking and baking as an economical alternative to reg-

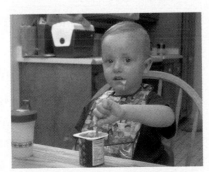

Fig. 12-9. Yogurt is a good source of calcium.

ular milk. If your loved one needs an extra source of protein and nourishment, powdered skim milk can be mixed with milk rather than water for puddings and milkshakes.

Fish, Poultry, Meat, Eggs, Dry Beans, and Nuts. These foods provide protein, minerals, and vitamins. In addition, meat is a good source of iron. Lower-fat choices from this group include most fish, chicken or turkey breast, lean cuts of meat, and dry beans. The Food Guide Pyramid suggests two to three servings from this group each day. One serving is two to three ounces of cooked meat, one egg, 1/2 cup cooked dry beans, or 1/3 cup of nuts.

Fats, Oils, and Sweets. Fats and oils help the body absorb fat-soluble vitamins. They also provide flavor and make us feel full. Fats are needed by the body in very small quantities. Most adults eat more fat than their bodies need. Fats contain more than twice as many calories per gram as carbohydrates or proteins. The body stores excess fat as fatty tissue. The best kinds of fats to use in a healthy diet are vegetable oils, including olive oil, canola oil, and corn oil (Fig 12-10). Sweets, including candy, cookies, cakes, pies, and ice cream, contain large amounts of fat and sugar. They should be eaten in much smaller amounts. In general, sweets have no nutritional value.

Some groups recommend a different Food Guide Pyramid for the elderly. It has a narrower base to reflect a decrease in energy needs. It emphasizes nutrient-dense

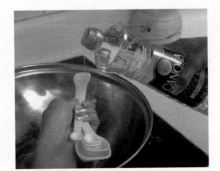

Fig. 12-10. Substitute olive, canola, or corn oil in recipes that call for less healthy oils.

foods, fiber, and water. Dietary supplements may be appropriate for many older people.

Due to slower metabolism and less activity, the elderly need to eat less to maintain body weight. Although calories can be reduced, daily needs for most vitamins and minerals do not decrease. Your loved one's doctor can help you understand these needs and recommend the best way to meet them.

Fluid Balance

As long as she is not on fluid restriction, your loved one should be encouraged to drink eight glasses, or 64 ounces, of water a day. As discussed above, water is essential for life (Fig. 12-11). Proper fluid intake is important; it helps prevent constipation and urinary incontinence. Without enough fluid, urine becomes concentrated, More concentrated urine creates a higher risk for infection. Proper fluid intake also helps to dilute wastes and flush out the urinary system. It may even help prevent confusion. Because the sense of thirst often diminishes as people age, any older person should be reminded to drink fluids often.

Dehydration occurs when a person does not have enough fluid in the body. People can become dehydrated not only from not drinking enough, but also if they are experiencing diarrhea or vomiting. Dehydration is a major problem

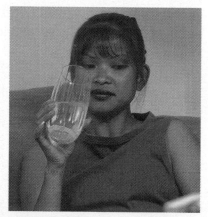

Fig. 12-11. A person who is not on a fluid restriction should drink 64 ounces of water per day.

among the elderly. Preventing dehydration is very important. Signs and symptoms of dehydration include the following:

- poor skin elasticity
- flushed, dry skin
- coated tongue
- decreased urine output
- confusion and irritability
- elevated body temperature
- decrease or absence of tears and/or saliva
- dry mouth
- cracked lips
- sunken eyes
- dark urine
- strong-smelling urine

GUIDELINES
Preventing Dehydration

Report observations and warning signs to your loved one's physician immediately.

Encourage your loved one to drink every time you see him.

Offer fresh water or other fluids often. Be aware of your loved one's preferences. He may like juice, water, or milk. Offer drinks that he enjoys. If he prefers drinks without ice, honor this preference.

If suggested by the doctor, record fluid intake and output.

Ice chips, frozen flavored ice sticks, and gelatin are also liquids. Offer them often. Do not offer ice chips or sticks if your loved one has a swallowing problem.

If appropriate, offer sips of liquid between bites of food at meals and snacks.

Make sure a pitcher and cup are close to your loved one and that they are light enough for him to lift.

Offer assistance if your loved one cannot drink without help. Use adaptive cups as needed.

To maintain health, the body must take in a certain amount of fluid each day. The fluid a person consumes is called intake, or input. When a person's intake is not in a healthy range, he can become dehydrated.

All fluid taken in each day cannot remain in the body. It must be eliminated as output. Output includes urine, feces, and vomitus. It also includes perspiration and moisture in the air exhaled. If a person's intake exceeds his or her output, the fluid is building up in body tissues. This fluid retention can cause medical problems and discomfort.

Fluid balance is maintaining equal intake and output. Most people regulate fluid balance automatically. But some people must have their intake and output, or I&O, monitored and documented (Fig. 12-12). To monitor this, you will need to measure and document all fluids your loved one takes by mouth as well as all urine and vomitus he produces.

Fluids are usually measured in cubic centimeters (cc). Ounces (oz) are converted to cubic centimeters. To convert ounces to cubic centimeters, multiply by 30.

Intake & Output Record

Client Name: _____ HHA Name: _____
Address: _____ Record Date: _____

Intake			Output		
Time	Type	Amount	Time	Urine Amount	Incontinent Episode

Output	Time	Approximate Amount
Vomiting		
Heavy Perspiration		
Diarrhea		

Fig. 12-12. A sample I&O sheet.

Conversions
A cubic centimeter is a unit of measure and is equal to one milliliter.

1 oz. = 30 cc or 30 ml.	7 oz. = 210 cc
2 oz. = 60 cc 3 oz. = 90 cc	8 oz. = 240 cc
4 oz. = 120 cc	¼ cup = 2 oz. = 60 cc
5 oz. = 150 cc	½ cup = 4 oz. = 120 cc
6 oz. = 1800 cc	1 cup = 8 oz. = 240 cc

Healthy Eating and Hydration

12

Measuring and recording intake and output

Equipment: I&O sheet, graduate (measuring container) (Fig. 12-13), pen and paper

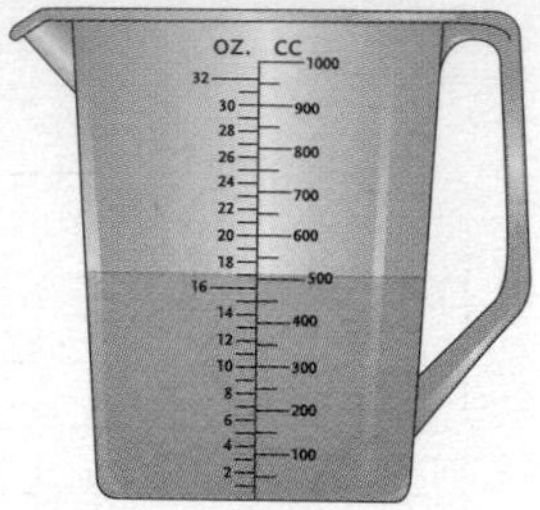

1 Wash hands.

2 Discuss what you will do.

3 Provide privacy.

Fig. 12-13. A graduate is a measuring container.

4 Using a graduate, measure the amount of fluid your loved one is served. Note the amount on paper.

5 When your loved one has finished a meal or snack, measure any leftover fluids. Note this amount on paper.

6 Subtract the leftover amount from the amount served. If you have measured in ounces, convert to cubic centimeters (cc) by multiplying by 30.

7 Document the amount of fluid consumed (in cc) in the input column on the I&O sheet. Record the time and what fluid was taken.

8 Wash your hands.

Measuring output is the other half of monitoring fluid balance.

Equipment: I&O sheet, graduate, gloves, pen and paper

1 Wash your hands.

2 Put on gloves before handling bedpan/urinal.

3 Pour the contents of the bedpan or urinal into measuring container without spilling or splashing any of the urine.

4 Measure the amount of urine while keeping container level.

5 After measuring urine, empty contents of measuring container into toilet without splashing.

6 Rinse measuring container and pour rinse water into toilet. Clean container.

7 Rinse bedpan/urinal and pour rinse water into toilet. Use disinfectant.

8 Return bedpan/urinal and measuring container to proper storage.

9 Remove and dispose of gloves.

10 Wash hands before recording output.

11 Record contents of container in output column on sheet.

Emesis, or vomiting, must be documented when monitoring intake and output. To measure vomitus, pour from basin into measuring container, then discard in the toilet. If your loved one vomits on the bed or floor, estimate the amount. Document emesis and amount on the I&O sheet.

Emesis may be a sign of illness or of a reaction to medication. Some people, such as cancer patients undergoing chemotherapy, may vomit frequently as a result of treatment. When your loved one vomits, check the color and consistency of vomitus. Look for blood in vomitus or blood-tinged vomitus. Report to the doctor and get instructions for diet. Vomiting is unpleasant. Handle it calmly and provide comfort to your loved one.

Fluid overload occurs when the body is unable to handle the amount of fluid consumed. This condition often affects people with heart or kidney disease. Signs and symptoms of fluid overload include the following:

- swelling/edema of extremities (ankles, feet, fingers, hands)

- weight gain (daily weight gain of one to two pounds)

- decreased urine output

- shortness of breath

- increased heart rate

- skin that appears tight, smooth, and shiny

If you suspect your loved one is experiencing either dehydration or fluid overload, contact your doctor.

Special Diets

If your loved one has an illness that affects certain organ systems, such as the heart, circulatory system, kidneys, liver, or pancreas, she may be placed on what is known as a "modified," "therapeutic," or "special" diet. Certain nutrients or fluids may be restricted or eliminated. Some medications may also interact with certain foods, which then must be restricted. If she has a nutritional deficiency, she may be placed on a special supplementary diet. Diets are also prescribed for weight control and food allergies.

As a caregiver, you play an essential role by ensuring that your loved one receives the basic nutrients essential to maintaining and improving her health while staying within the dietary modifications prescribed.

Sodium-Restricted Diet (Low-Sodium Diet). People are most familiar with sodium as one of the two ingredients of salt. Salt is the first food to be restricted in a low-sodium diet because it is high in sodium.

Excess sodium causes the body to retain more water in tissues and in the circulatory system than is necessary. This causes the heart to pump harder, a situation that is harmful for people who have high blood pressure, coronary artery disease, or kidney disease. A modified fluid intake may also be required for people with these conditions, because too much fluid can lead to congestive heart failure.

The human body needs 1,500 to 2,500 milligrams of sodium a day; however, on average, we consume twice that amount. Excess sodium is excreted in the urine and, over the years, can erode the kidneys, leading to hypertension and kidney disease.

Foods high in sodium include the following:

- cured meats: ham, bacon, lunchmeat, sausage, salt pork, and hot dogs

- salty or smoked fish: herring, salted cod, sardines, anchovies, caviar, smoked salmon or lox

- processed cheese

- canned and dried soups

- vegetables preserved in brine: pickles, sauerkraut, olives, relishes

- salted foods: nuts, dips, and spreads

- sauces and condiments with high concentrations of salt: Worcestershire, barbecue, chili, and soy sauces; ketchup and mustard

- canned foods

- some cereals

- over-the-counter medications and drugs

Read product labels to determine if they contain salt or sodium in any form. Common forms of sodium include monosodium glutamate, often added to meat tenderizers, seasonings, and prepared foods to enhance flavor; and sodium nitrate, a salt used to preserve lunchmeats and other cured meats.

You can make low-sodium meals more flavorful by adding lemon, herbs, dry mustard, pepper, paprika, orange rind, onion, and garlic to recipes. The flavor of meats can also be enhanced by the addition of fruits and jellies. Salt substitutes should only be used with the doctor's approval. These seasonings might be high in potassium, a substance that is harmful to people with certain illnesses, such as kidney disease.

Fluid-Restricted Diets. The amount of fluid taken into the body through food and fluids must equal the amount of fluid that leaves the body through perspiration, stool, urine, and expiration. This is fluid balance. When fluid intake is greater than fluid output, body tissues become swollen with excess fluid. In addition, people with severe heart disease and kidney disease may have difficulty processing large volumes of fluid. To prevent further heart and kidney damage, doctors may restrict a person's fluid intake. If your loved one is on fluid restriction, you will need to measure and document exact amounts of fluid intake.

High Potassium Diets (K+). If your loved one is on diuretics, which are medications that reduce fluid volume, or on some blood pressure medications, he may be excreting so much fluid that his body could be depleted of potassium. Or he may be placed on a high potassium diet for a different reason.

Foods high in potassium include bananas, grapefruit, oranges, orange juice, prune juice, prunes, dried apricots, figs, raisins, dates, cantaloupes, tomatoes, potatoes with skins, sweet potatoes and yams, winter squash, legumes, avocados, and unsalted nuts.

Low-Protein Diet. In addition to restricted dietary intake of fluids, sodium, and potassium, people who have kidney disease may also be on low-protein diets. Protein is restricted because it breaks down into compounds that may lead to further kidney damage. The extent of the restriction depends on the stage of the disease and whether the person is on dialysis.

Exchange lists show foods that can be exchanged for one another in a meal plan. They are used extensively in special diets for people with diabetes. However, exchange lists have also been developed for those on diets modified for protein, potassium, and sodium.

Low-Fat/Low-Cholesterol Diet. People who have high levels of cholesterol in their blood are at risk for heart attacks and other heart disease. People with gallbladder disease, diseases that interfere with fat digestion, and liver disease are also placed on low-fat/low-cholesterol diets.

Low-fat/low-cholesterol diets permit skim milk, low-fat cottage cheese, fish, white meat of turkey and chicken, veal, and vegetable fats, especially monounsaturated fats such as olive, canola, and peanut oils (Fig. 12-14). People on low-fat/low-cholesterol diets may be advised to limit their diets in the following ways:

- Eat lean cuts of meat including lamb, beef, and pork; limit even these to three times a week.

- Limit egg yolks to three or four per week, including eggs used in baking.

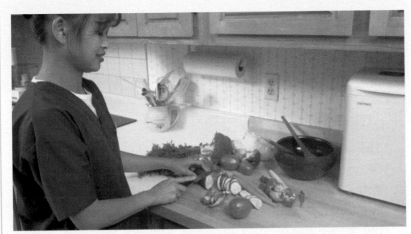

Fig. 12-14. Vegetables are an important component of a low-fat/low-cholesterol diet.

- Avoid organ meats, shellfish, fatty meats, cream, butter, lard, meat drippings, coconut and palm oils, and desserts and soups made with whole milk.

- Avoid fried foods and sweets.

People who have gallbladder disease or other digestive problems may be placed on a diet that restricts all fats.

Modified Calorie Diet for Weight Management. Some people need to reduce calories to lose weight or prevent additional weight gain. Others may need to gain weight and increase calories because of malnutrition, surgery, illness, or fever. Those with certain conditions may need to increase protein intake to promote growth and repair of tissue and regulation of body functions.

Dietary Management of Ulcers. Gastric and duodenal ulcers can be irritated by foods that produce or increase levels of acid in the stomach. People who have ulcers usually know the foods that cause them discomfort. Doctors will advise them to avoid

these foods as well as alcohol; beverages containing caffeine, such as coffee, tea, and soft drinks; and spicy seasonings such as black pepper, cayenne, and chili pepper. Three meals or more a day are usually advised. If alcohol is allowed, it should be drunk with meals.

Dietary Management of Diabetes Mellitus. Calories and carbohydrates are carefully regulated in the dietary management of diabetes (Fig. 12-15). Protein and fats are also regulated. The types of foods and the amounts consumed are determined by the person's nutritional and energy requirements. Two types of diets can manage diabetes:

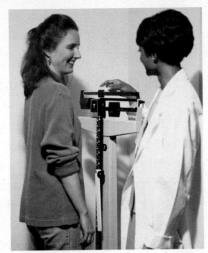

Fig. 12-15. Diabetics must be careful about what they eat as well as their weight.

1. **Non-concentrated Sweets Diet.** This diet is a regular, well-balanced diet that excludes concentrated sweets, such as sugars, honey, syrup, jellies, jams, preserves, candy, and cranberry sauce (Fig. 12-16). This diet also eliminates cakes, pastries, cookies, puddings, ice cream, gel-

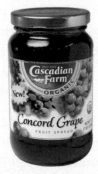

Fig. 12-16. Jellies, jams, and preserves are excluded from a non-concentrated sweets diet.

atin, sweetened fruit juices and beverages, sugar-coated cereals, condensed milk, and candied or glazed fruits and vegetables.

2. **Exchange List Diets**. Exchange list diets are described in more detail in the discussion of diabetes found in chapter 7. This type of diet is more restricted than the non-concentrated sweets diet, because it involves more than just the elimination of concentrated sweets. Meals are carefully planned based on exact amounts of food from the six food groups. Exchange lists are then used to determine foods and the exact serving sizes that may be eaten to follow the meal plan. Foods are measured and must be eaten completely at certain times. Eating the necessary carbohydrates, which are found in dairy and bread groups, is very important if the person is too ill to tolerate the other foods. Any variation in eating patterns and routine must be reported to the physician or nurse.

Liquid Diets. A liquid diet is made up of foods that are liquid at body temperature. Liquid diets are usually ordered as "clear" or "full." A clear liquid diet includes clear juices, broth, gelatin, and popsicles. A full liquid diet includes clear liquids with the addition of cream soups, milk and ice cream. A liquid diet is usually ordered for a short time. It may be ordered due to a medical condition or before or after a test or surgery.

Soft Diet. The soft diet is soft in texture. It consists of soft or chopped foods that are easier to chew and swallow. Doctors order this diet for people who have trouble chewing and swallowing due to dental problems or other medical conditions.

Pureed Diet. To puree a food means to chop, blend, or grind it into a thick paste of baby food consistency. The food should be thick enough to hold its form in the mouth. This diet does not need to be chewed. A pureed diet is often used for people who have trouble chewing and/or swallowing more textured foods.

Thickened Liquids. People with swallowing problems may be restricted to consuming only thickened liquids. Thickening improves the ability to control fluid in the mouth and throat. A doctor orders the necessary thickness after the person has been evaluated by a speech therapist. Special products are used for thickening. If thickening is ordered, it must be used with all liquids. Do not offer regular liquids, including water, to a person who is on a diet of thickened liquids.

Three basic thickened consistencies are:

1. **Nectar Thick**: This consistency is thicker than water. It is the thickness of a thick juice, such as pear nectar or tomato juice. A person can drink liquids of this thickness from a cup.

2. **Honey Thick**: This consistency has the thickness of honey. It will pour very slowly. A person will usually use a spoon to consume it.

3. **Pudding Thick**: With this consistency, the liquids have become semi-solid, much like pudding. A spoon should stand up straight in the glass when put into the middle of the drink. A person must consume these liquids with a spoon.

When a person is too ill to receive adequate nutrition by mouth, artificial feeding becomes necessary. Chapter 11 has information on artificial feeding and feeding tubes.

Safe Food Preparation

Food-borne illnesses affect up to 100 million people each year. Elderly people are at increased risk partly because they may not see, smell, or taste that food is spoiled. They also may not have the energy to prepare and store food safely. For people who have weakened immune systems because of AIDS or cancer, a food-borne illness can be deadly. Remember the following guidelines for safe food preparation:

GUIDELINES
Safe Food Preparation

Wash hands frequently. Wash your hands thoroughly before beginning any food preparation. Wash your hands after handling raw meat, poultry, or fish.

Keep everything clean. Clean and disinfect countertops and other surfaces before, during (as necessary), and after food preparation.

Handle raw meat, poultry and fish carefully. Use an antibacterial kitchen cleaner or a diluted bleach solution to clean any countertops on which meat juices are spilled. Wrap paper or packaging containing meat juices in plastic and discard immediately.

Once you have used a knife or cutting board to cut raw meat, do not use it for anything else until it has been washed in the dishwasher or in very hot, soapy water containing bleach. Use plastic cutting boards for raw meat and wooden ones for vegetables and other foods (Fig. 12-17).

Change dishcloths, sponges and towels frequently. Sponges may be washed in the dishwasher to disinfect them.

Defrost frozen foods in the refrigerator, not on the countertop. Do not remove meats or dairy products from the refrigerator until just before use.

Wash fruits and vegetables thoroughly in running water to remove pesticides and bacteria.

Cook meats, poultry, and fish thoroughly to kill any harmful microorganisms they may contain (Fig. 12-18). Heat leftovers thoroughly. Never leave food out for over two hours. Keep cold foods cold and hot foods hot.

To store food safely, follow these tips:

- Buy cold food last, and get it home fast. After shopping, put away refrigerated foods first.

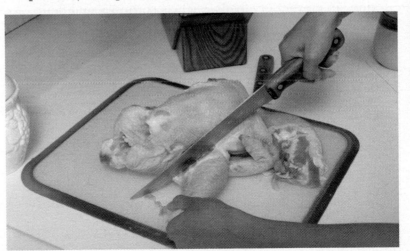

Fig. 12-17. Use plastic cutting boards for raw meat.

Healthy Eating and Hydration

12

• Keep it safe—refrigerate. Maintain refrigerator temperature between 36° F and 40° F; maintain freezer temperature at 0° F. Refrigerated items that spoil easily should be kept in the rear of the refrigerator, not the door.

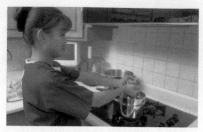

Fig. 12-18. Cook foods thoroughly to kill microorganisms.

Look on the jar or package to determine whether a food item requires refrigeration once it has been opened (Fig.12-19). Salad dressings, mayonnaise, and other items with fat in them require refrigeration after they have been opened. Do not refreeze items after they have been thawed.

• Use small containers that seal tightly. Foods cool more quickly when stored in smaller containers. Never leave foods out for more than two hours. Tightly cover all foods and store with enough room around them for air circulation. To prevent dry foods, such as cornmeal and flour, from becoming infested with insects, store these items in

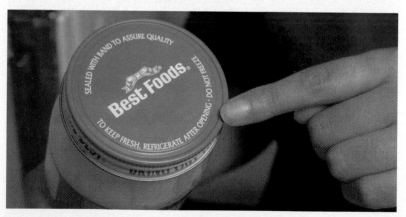

Fig. 12-19. Look for refrigeration guidelines on food labels.

tightly sealed containers. If you find items that are already infested, discard them and use a clean container to store a fresh supply.

• When in doubt, throw it out! If you are not sure whether food is spoiled, do not take any chances. Discard it. Check the expiration dates on foods, especially perishables. Check the refrigerator frequently for spoiled foods and discard any you find.

Assisting with Eating

If your loved one needs help to feed herself, she may become depressed or embarrassed about her dependence on you. Be sensitive to her feelings. Only give assistance when necessary or when she requests it. Encourage her to do whatever she can for herself. For example, if she can hold and use a napkin, she should. Try adaptive utensils to allow her to remain independent for as long as possible.

Just like dehydration, unintended weight loss is a serious problem for the elderly. Weight loss can mean that a person has a serious medical condition, and it can lead to skin breakdown. This leads to pressure sores. If your loved one is losing weight, report it to the doctor, no matter how small the amount. Diabetes, chronic obstructive pulmonary disease, cancer, HIV, and other diseases put a person at a greater risk for malnutrition.

GUIDELINES
Preventing Unintended Weight Loss

Encourage your loved one to eat. Talk about food served in a positive tone of voice and with positive words.

Honor her food likes and dislikes.

Offer different kinds of foods and beverages.

Help her if she has trouble feeding herself.

Make food look, taste, and smell good. She may have a poor sense of taste and smell.

Season foods according to her preferences, even pureed foods.

Allow time for her to finish eating.

If she has trouble using utensils, report it to the doctor. Many kinds of adaptive aids can assist with eating (Fig. 12-20).

Record meal/snack intake.

Give oral care before and after meals.

Position your loved one sitting upright for eating.

If she has had a loss of appetite and/or seems sad, ask about it.

Check to make sure that her dentures fit properly.

Report any difficulty with chewing and swallowing or mouth pain to the doctor.

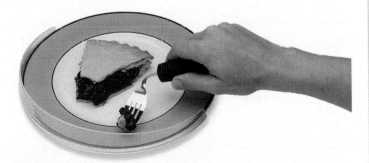

Fig. 12-20. Types of adaptive devices for eating. (Photo courtesy of North Coast Medical, Inc. www.ncmedical.com, 800-821-9319)

Assisting someone with eating

Equipment: meal, eating utensils, clothing protector, if appropriate, 1–2 napkins or washcloths

1 Wash your hands.

2 Explain what you will do.

3 Provide privacy as needed.

4 Assist your loved one to wash her hands if she cannot do it on her own.

5 See that she is in an upright sitting position (at a 90-degree angle).

6 Assist her to put on a clothing protector, if desired.

7 Sit next to your loved one at her eye level (Fig.12-21). Sit on her stronger side if she has one-sided weakness.

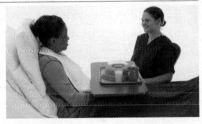

Fig. 12-21.

8 Check temperature of food. Offer the food in bite-sized pieces (Fig. 12-22). Alternate types of food offered, allowing for your loved one's preferences, i.e. do not feed all of one type of food before offering another type. Make sure her mouth

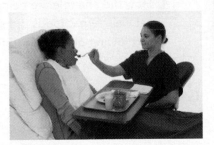

Fig. 12-22.

is empty before offering the next bite of food or sip of drink.

9   Offer drinks throughout the meal. If you are holding the cup, touch it to her lips before you tip it. Give small, frequent sips. She may prefer to use a straw or an adaptive cup. Training cups are an inexpensive way to make it easier for your loved one to drink by herself.

10   Wipe food from her mouth and hands as necessary during the meal. Wipe again at the end of the meal (Fig. 12-23).

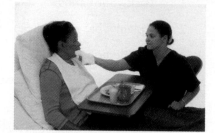

Fig. 12-23.

11   Talk with your loved one during the meal. It makes mealtime more enjoyable. Do not rush her.

12   When she is done eating, remove the clothing protector if used. Remove the tray or dishes.

13   Wash your hands.

14   Assist your loved one in leaving the table or shifting to a comfortable position.

15   Document her intake if required, and any observations. How did she tolerate being upright for the meal? Did she eat well? What foods did she eat or not eat? Report any swallowing difficulties to the doctor.

Resources

The USDA has information about food safety, dietary health, and food labeling and packaging. There is also a list of food recalls and information on food technology. The USDA offers dietary plans for people on a budget and a wealth of information about the Food Guide Pyramid, which was developed by the USDA.

U.S. Department of Agriculture (USDA)
Food and Nutrition Page
1400 Independence Ave.
S.W. Washington, DC 20250
www.usda.gov

The Nutrition.gov site contains information on healthy eating, nutrition, and obesity prevention.

Nutrition.gov
National Agricultural Library
Food and Nutrition Information Center
Nutrition.gov Staff
10301 Baltimore Avenue
Beltsville, MD 20705-2351
www.nutrition.gov

Emergency Care

Medical emergencies may be the result of accidents or sudden illnesses. In this chapter you will learn how to respond appropriately to medical emergencies. Heart attacks, strokes, diabetic emergencies, choking, automobile accidents, and gunshot wounds are all medical emergencies. Falls, burns, and cuts can also be emergencies when they are severe.

First Steps

Familiarize yourself with basic emergency care procedures. Check with your physician to find out if there are certain kinds of emergencies, such as seizures or fainting, that you should be especially alert and prepared for due to your loved one's condition.

If you are not already trained to perform CPR, contact your local branch of the American Red Cross or American Heart Association and find out when and where CPR classes are offered. Make an effort to keep your certification current.

Prepare yourself and your household in advance for any unforeseen emergencies. Assemble a disaster emergency kit (see the last section of this chapter) and make sure everyone in the home knows where it is stored. Make an evacuation plan for use in case of emergency and make sure everyone in the home is familiar with it. Find out which disasters are likely to occur in your area and make a plan and procure supplies to respond in case they occur.

In an emergency situation, it is important to remain calm, act quickly, and communicate clearly. Memorizing the following steps will help you respond calmly and quickly in an emergency:

Assess the situation. Try to determine what has happened. Make sure you are not in danger. Notice the time.

Assess the victim. Ask the injured or ill person what has happened. If the person is unable to respond, he may be unconscious. To determine whether a person is conscious, tap the person and ask if he is all right. Speak loudly and use his name. If there is no response, assume the person is unconscious and that you have an emergency situation. Call for help right away or send someone else to call.

If a person is conscious and able to speak, then he is breathing and has a pulse. Talk with him about what happened, and check him for injury. Look for the following:

- severe bleeding

- changes in consciousness

- irregular breathing

- unusual color or feel to the skin

- swollen places on the body

- medical alert tags

- anything the person says is painful

If one of these conditions exists, you may need professional medical help.

If the injured or ill person is conscious, he may feel panic about his condition. Listen to the person. Tell him what actions are being taken to help him. Be calm and confident to reassure him that he is being taken care of.

Most emergencies will require that you or someone nearby call for emergency assistance immediately. Always have an emergency phone list near the telephone. Throughout this chapter, you will learn procedures for assisting in various emergencies. Each procedure includes instructions on when to call for help.

Reporting Emergencies

When in doubt about calling for help, call! If you need to call emergency medical services, call 911 or dial 0 for the operator. If you are alone, make the call yourself. If you are not alone, shout for help and have someone else make the call and then return to you.

When calling emergency services, be prepared to give the following information:

- the phone number and address of the emergency, including exact directions or landmarks if necessary

- the person's condition, including any medical background you know

- your name and relationship to the victim

- details of any first aid being given

The dispatcher you speak with may need other information or may want to give you other instructions. Do not hang up the phone until the dispatcher hangs up or tells you to hang up. If you are in a home, unlock the front door so emergency personnel can get in when they arrive.

If the person is breathing, has a normal pulse, is normally responsive, and is not bleeding severely, you may not need to call for emergency services. If your loved one has fallen, been burned, or cut himself but the damage seems to be minor, call his doctor. Let the person answering the phone know that an accident has occurred. Try to remember as many details as possible, and remember to report the facts only.

First Aid Procedures

First aid is care given in an emergency before trained medical professionals can take over. Cardiopulmonary resuscitation (CPR) refers to medical procedures used when a person's heart or lungs have stopped working. CPR is used until medical help arrives. Quick action is necessary. CPR must be started immediately. Brain damage may occur within four to six minutes after the heart stops beating and the lungs stop breathing. The person can die within 10 minutes.

Only properly trained people should administer CPR; it is a good idea to get this training. Training is usually offered by the American Heart Association or the Red Cross. Look in your phone book or on the Internet for local numbers to find out when and where classes are offered. If you are trained and you have a current card, perform CPR when needed in an emergency. If you are not trained, do not attempt to perform CPR (Fig. 13-1). Performing CPR incorrectly can further injure a person; for example, delivering chest compressions in the wrong place can result in a punctured lung.

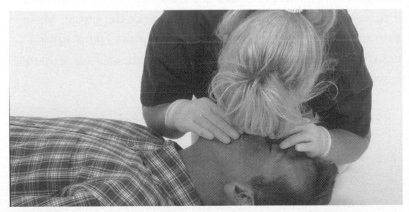

Fig. 13-1. Do not attempt to perform CPR unless you have been trained.

Choking

People who have difficulty chewing or swallowing, are confused, or have poor vision may be at risk of choking. When something is blocking the tube through which air enters the lungs, the person has an obstructed airway. When people are choking, they usually put their hands to their throats and cough (Fig. 13-2). As long as the

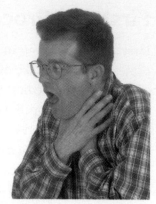

Fig. 13-2. When a person is choking, he will usually put his hands to his throat and cough.

person can speak, breathe, or cough, do nothing. Encourage him to cough as forcefully as possible to get the object out. Stay with the person at all times, until he stops choking or can no longer speak, breathe, or cough. Do not hit him on the back.

If a person can no longer speak, breathe, or cough, call 911 immediately. After calling 911 return to the person. The Heimlich maneuver is a procedure used for choking. It uses abdominal thrusts to move the blockage upward, out of the throat. Make sure the person needs help before starting the Heimlich maneuver. If the person cannot speak or cough, or if his response is weak, start the Heimlich maneuver.

Heimlich maneuver for the conscious person

1   Stand behind the person and bring your arms under his arms. Wrap your arms around his waist.

2   Make a fist with one hand. Place the flat, thumb side of

the fist against the person's abdomen, above the navel but below the breastbone.

3   Grasp the fist with your other hand. Pull both hands toward you and up, quickly and forcefully (Fig. 13-3).

4   Repeat until the object is pushed out or the person loses consciousness.

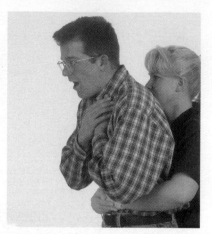

Fig. 13-3.

If the person becomes unconscious, help him to the floor gently. Lie him on his back with his face up. Make sure help is on its way. He may have a completely blocked airway. He needs professional medical help immediately.

Shock

Shock occurs when organs and tissues in the body do not receive an adequate blood supply. Bleeding, heart attack, severe infection, and conditions that cause the blood pressure to fall can lead to shock. Shock can become worse when the person is extremely frightened or in severe pain.

Shock is a dangerous, life-threatening situation. Signs of shock include pale or bluish skin, staring, increased pulse and respiration rates, decreased blood pressure, and extreme thirst. Always call for emergency help if you suspect a person is experiencing shock. To prevent or treat shock, do the following:

Shock

1   Have the person lie down on her back. If the person is bleeding from the mouth or vomiting, place her on her side (unless you suspect that the neck, back, or spinal cord is injured).

2   Control bleeding. This procedure is described later in the chapter.

3   Check pulse and respirations if possible.

4   Keep the person as calm and comfortable as possible.

5   Maintain normal body temperature. If the weather is cold, place a blanket around the person. If the weather is hot, provide shade.

6   Elevate the feet unless the person has a head or abdominal injury, breathing difficulties, or a fractured bone or back (Fig. 13-4). Elevate the head and shoulders if a head wound or breathing difficulties are present. Never elevate a body part if a broken bone exists.

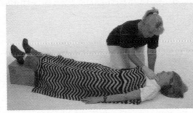

Fig. 13-4

7   Do not give the person anything to eat or drink.

8   Call for emergency help immediately. Victims of shock should always receive medical care as soon as possible.

Myocardial Infarction or Heart Attack

Myocardial infarction, or heart attack, occurs when the heart muscle does not receive enough oxygen because blood vessels are blocked. Signs of a heart attack include the following:

- sudden, severe pain in the chest, usually on the left side or in the center, behind the breastbone

- indigestion or heartburn

- nausea and vomiting

- dyspnea, or difficulty breathing

- dizziness

- pale, gray, or bluish (cyanotic) skin color, indicating lack of oxygen

- perspiration

- cold and clammy skin

- weak and irregular pulse rate

- low blood pressure

- anxiety and a sense of doom

- denial of a heart problem

The pain of a heart attack is commonly described as a crushing, pressing, squeezing, stabbing, piercing pain, or "like someone is sitting on my chest." The pain may go down the inside of the left arm. A person may also feel it in the neck and/or in the jaw. The pain usually does not go away. You must take immediate action if a person has any of these symptoms. Follow these steps:

Heart attack

1   Call or have someone call emergency services, and call the doctor.

2   Place the person in a comfortable position. Encourage him to rest, and reassure him that you will not leave him alone.

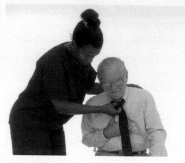

3   Loosen clothing around the neck (Fig. 13-5).

Fig. 13-5.

4   Do not give the person liquids.

5   If the person takes heart medication, such as nitroglycerin, find the medication and offer it.

6   Monitor breathing and pulse. If the person stops breathing or has no pulse, perform rescue breathing or CPR if you are trained to do so.

7   Stay with the person until help arrives.

Bleeding

Severe bleeding can cause death quickly and must be controlled. Call for help immediately, then follow these steps to control bleeding:

Bleeding

1   Put on gloves.

2   Hold a thick sterile pad, a clean pad, or a clean cloth such as a handkerchief or towel against the wound. Have the injured person use his bare hand until you can get a clean pad. Also have the person hold the pad, if he is able, until you can put on gloves.

3   Press down hard directly on the bleeding wound until help arrives. Do not decrease pressure (Fig. 13-6). **Fig. 13-6.**

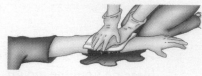

Put additional pads over the first pad if blood seeps through. Do not remove the first pad.

4   Raise the wound above the heart to slow down the bleeding. If the wound is on an arm, leg, hand, or foot, and there are no broken bones, prop up the limb on towels, blankets, coats, or other absorbent material.

5   When bleeding is under control, secure the dressing to keep it in place. Check the person for symptoms of shock (pale skin, increased pulse and respiration rates, decreased blood pressure, and extreme thirst). Stay with the person until medical help arrives.

6   Wash hands thoroughly when finished.

Poisoning

First aid kits in the home should contain syrup of ipecac, activated charcoal, and Epsom salts for the treatment of accidental poisoning (Fig. 13-7). Always have the poison control center phone number available. Suspect poisoning when a person suddenly collapses, vomits, and has heavy, labored breathing. If you suspect poisoning, take the following steps:

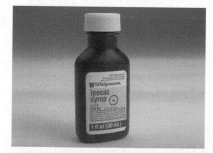

Fig. 13-7. Ipecac syrup causes vomiting and should only be used when directed by a doctor or a poison control center.

Poisoning

1   Look for a container that will help you determine what the person has taken or eaten. Check the mouth for chemical burns and note the breath odor.

2   Call the local or state poison control center immediately. Follow instructions from poison control.

3   Notify the doctor.

Burns

Care of a burn depends on its depth, size, and location. There are three types of burns: first-degree, second-degree, and third-degree burns (Fig. 13-8).

First-degree burns involve just the epidermis, or outer layer of skin. The skin becomes red, painful, and swollen, but no blisters occur. Second-degree burns extend from the outer layer of the skin to the next deeper layer of skin, the dermis. The skin is red, painful, swollen, and blisters occur. Third-degree burns involve all three layers of the skin and may extend to the bone. If the nerves are destroyed, no pain occurs. The skin is shiny and appears hard. It may be white in color.

You should call for emergency help in any of the following situations:

- An infant or child, or an

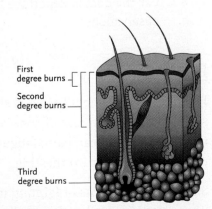

First degree burns
Second degree burns
Third degree burns

Fig. 13-8.

elderly, ill or weak person has been burned, unless the burn is very minor.

- The burn occurs on the head, neck, hands, feet, face, or genitals, or burns cover more than one body part.

- The person who has been burned is having trouble breathing.

- The burn was caused by chemicals, electricity, or an explosion.

Burns

To treat a minor burn:

1   Use cool, clean water (not ice) to decrease the skin temperature and prevent further injury (Fig. 13-9). Ice will cause further skin damage. Dampen a clean cloth and place it over the burn.

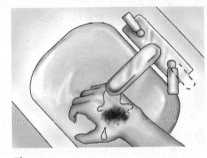

Fig. 13-9.

2   Once the pain has eased, you may cover the area with dry, sterile gauze.

3   Never use any kind of ointment, salve, or grease on a burn.

For more serious burns:

1   Remove the person from the source of the burn. If clothing has caught fire, smother it with a blanket or towel to extinguish flames. Protect yourself from the source of the burn.

2   Check for breathing, pulse, and severe bleeding.

3   Call for emergency help.

4   Do not apply water. It may cause infection.

5   Remove as much of the person's clothing around the burned area as possible, but do not try to pull away clothing that sticks to the burn. Cover the burn with a thick, dry, sterile gauze if available, or a clean cloth. A dry, insulated cool pack may be used over the dressing (Fig. 13-10). Again, never use any kind of ointment, salve, or grease on a burn.

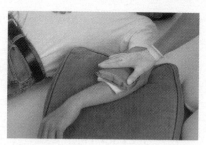

Fig. 13-10.

6   Ask the person to lie down and elevate the affected part if this does not cause greater pain.

7   If the burn covers a large area, wrap the person or the limb in a dry, clean sheet. Take care not to rub the skin.

8   Wait for emergency medical help.

Seizures

Seizures are involuntary, often violent, contractions of muscles. They can involve a small area or the entire body. Seizures are caused by an abnormality in the brain. They can occur in young children who have a high fever. Older children and adults who have a serious illness, fever, head injury, or a seizure disorder such as epilepsy may also have convulsions.

The primary goal of a caregiver during a seizure is to make sure the person is safe. During a seizure, a person may shake severely, thrust arms and legs uncontrollably, clench his jaw, drool, and be unable to swallow. The following emergency measures should be taken if a person has a seizure:

Seizures

1   Lower the person to the floor.

2   Have someone call for emergency medical help if needed. Do not leave the person during the seizure unless you must do so to get medical help.

3   Move furniture away to prevent injury. If a pillow is nearby, place it under the person's head.

4   Do not try to restrain the person.

5   Do not force anything between the person's teeth. Do not place your hands in the person's mouth for any reason. You could be severely bitten.

6   Do not give liquids.

7   When the seizure is over, check breathing.

8   Call the doctor. Report the length of the seizure and your observations.

Fainting

Fainting occurs when the blood supply to the brain drops, resulting in a sudden loss of consciousness. Fainting may be the result of hunger, fear, pain, fatigue, standing for a long time, poor ventilation, or overheating.

Signs and symptoms of fainting include dizziness, perspiration, pale skin, weak pulse, shallow respirations, and blackness in the visual field. If someone appears likely to faint, follow these steps:

Fainting

1. Have the person lie down or sit down before fainting occurs.

2. If the person is in a sitting position, have her bend forward and place her head between her knees (Fig. 13-11). If the person is lying flat on her back, elevate the legs.

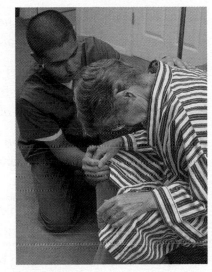

3. Loosen any tight clothing.

4. Have the person stay in position for at least five minutes after symptoms disappear.

Fig. 13-11.

5. Help the person get up slowly and continue to observe her for symptoms of fainting.

6. Call the doctor and report the incident.

If a person does faint, lower her to the floor or other flat surface. Position her on her back. Elevate her legs 8 to 12 inches, and loosen any tight clothing. Check to make sure she is breathing. She should recover quickly, but keep her lying down for several minutes. Call the doctor immediately. Fainting may be a sign of a more serious medical condition.

Nosebleed

A nosebleed can occur spontaneously, when the air is dry, or when injury has occurred. The medical term for a nosebleed is "epistaxis." If a person has a nosebleed, take the following steps:

Nosebleed

1. Elevate the head of the bed or tell the person to remain in a sitting position. Offer tissues or a clean cloth to catch the blood. Do not touch blood or bloody clothes, tissues or cloths without gloves.

2. Put on gloves. Apply firm pressure over the bridge of the nose. Squeeze the bridge of the nose with your thumb and forefinger (Fig. 13-12). Have the person do this until you are able to get gloves on.

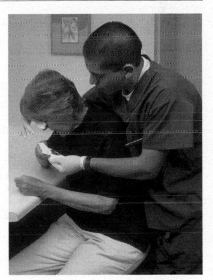

3. Apply the pressure consistently until the bleeding stops.

4. Use a cool cloth or ice wrapped in a cloth on the back of the neck, the forehead, or the upper lip to slow the flow of blood. Never apply ice directly to skin.

Fig. 13-12.

5. Report the nosebleed to the doctor.

Falls

Falls can be minor or severe. All falls should be reported to a doctor. In the case of a severe fall, call emergency medical services immediately. Take the following steps to help someone who has fallen:

Helping someone who has fallen

1	Assess the person's condition. Determine if she is unconscious, not breathing, has no pulse, or is bleeding severely. Get emergency medical help if any of these conditions exist.
2	Look for broken bones. Pain and body parts lying in an unnatural position or bones protruding through the skin are indications.
3	If the person seems unhurt, encourage her to stay down until you can check her condition thoroughly.
4	Ask her to move each body part separately to be sure there are no strains, sprains, or fractures.
5	If you find no evidence of injury, make her as comfortable as possible.
6	Call the doctor and report the fall immediately.

See chapter 4 for more information on falls.

Emergency Evacuations

If a fire or other disaster occurs, you may need to get yourself, your loved one, and other members of the household out of the home immediately. Leaving in an emergency is called evacuation. Because you may not have a lot of time to think or plan in an emergency, you should know in advance how best to evacuate your home.

Plan for evacuation by doing the following:

- Locate all the doors and windows that could serve as exits in an emergency.

- In an apartment building, know where fire stairs are located. Elevators may be unsafe in an emergency.

- Know the location of disaster supplies, including fire extinguishers, ladders for escape from upper floors, first aid kits or supplies, and utility shut-off points.

- Discuss a plan for evacuation with your loved one and other family members. Emphasize that everyone should keep calm in an emergency.

- Know who will be responsible for helping infants, children, and the disabled in emergencies.

- Agree on a place outside the home for everyone to meet after evacuation.

Disaster Procedures

Disasters can include fire, flood, earthquake, hurricane, tornado, or severe weather. The disasters you may experience will depend on where you live. Know the appropriate action to take to protect yourself and your loved one. If you live in an area that is prone to disasters, call the local chapter of the Red Cross to learn more about how to prepare for and handle disasters.

The following guidelines apply in any disaster situation:

- Remain calm.

- Listen to radio or television bulletins to keep informed. A battery-powered radio will help you to stay informed if the power goes out.

- If a disaster, such as a tornado or hurricane, is forecast, be ready. Wear appropriate clothing and shoes. Have family members dressed and ready in case evacuation is necessary.

- Stay in contact with others if possible. Let someone know where you are, what conditions are, and where you will go if you must evacuate.

- Locate disaster supplies. Ideally, a disaster supply kit should be assembled before disaster strikes.

Emergency Supplies

Keep enough supplies in your home to meet your needs for at least three days. Assemble a disaster supply kit with items you may need in an evacuation. Store these supplies in sturdy, easy-to-carry containers such as backpacks, duffel bags or covered trash containers. Include:

- A three-day supply of water (one gallon per person per day) and food that won't spoil.

- One change of clothing and footwear per person, and one blanket or sleeping bag per person.

- A first aid kit that includes your family's prescription medications.

- Emergency tools, including a battery-powered radio, flashlight, and plenty of extra batteries.

- An extra set of car keys and a credit card, cash, or traveler's checks.

- Sanitation supplies.

- Special items for infant, elderly, or disabled family members.

- An extra pair of glasses.

- Important family documents in a waterproof container.

Resources

The American Red Cross provides disaster services and health and safety services. Their site has disaster preparation tips, news of worldwide relief efforts, and links for those wishing to contribute to relief efforts or to give blood.

American Red Cross
American Red Cross National Headquarters
2025 E Street, NW
Washington, DC 20006
Tel: 202-303-4498
Disaster Assistance: 866-GET-INFO (866-438-4636)
www.redcross.org

The American Heart Association offers information on heart health and heart diseases and conditions. Their site provides a link that allows you to find your local AHA branch.

American Heart Association
National Center
7272 Greenville Avenue
Dallas, TX 75231
Tel: 800-AHA-USA-1 or 800-242-8721
www.americanheart.org

Medications

One of the most intimidating aspects of caring for a loved one in your home is the management of medications. Many older adults take multiple medications, prescribed by different doctors, to manage several long-term illnesses at once. Your loved one is also probably taking some over-the-counter medications as well. Under these conditions, it is easy for medications to become the major focus of your day, every day (Fig. 14-1). It can be a difficult task, but it is not an unmanageable one.

This chapter offers some tools to help you keep track of and manage your loved one's medications. It will help you learn what to watch for and what to report to the doctor and pharmacist. It will not contain all of the answers, but you will not be expected to know all of the answers. What you do need to know is which information is valuable and needs to be reported to your loved one's physician.

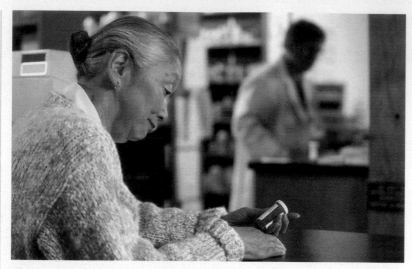

Fig. 14-1. Many older adults take multiple medications.

First Steps

Make a list of all of the doctors and pharmacies used by your loved one.

Make a list of all medications he is taking. Include all herbs, vitamins, supplements, and over-the-counter medications he takes. Include a list of all allergies and adverse reactions to medication that he has experienced. Remember to take this list to all medical appointments, consultations, and trips to the emergency room.

Designate a primary physician to keep track of all medications being taken at a given time.

Consult this physician to make sure that all of the medications your loved one is taking are safe to use together; do this as often as needed when treatments change.

Medications and Older Adults

One important thing to remember is that drugs behave differently in the bodies of older adults than in younger adults. Chronic illnesses as well as the normal changes of aging can affect the way drugs are absorbed and metabolized in the body. As people age, their ratio of body fat to muscle increases. As many drugs are stored in the fat cells, this increase can cause drugs to build up more quickly in the bodies of older adults. Reduced metabolism and less efficient function of the liver and kidneys also allow drugs to remain in the body longer. Dehydration can cause drugs to become concentrated in the body.

While people over the age of 65 use more prescription and over-the-counter drugs than any other age group in the United States, drug research and trials are typically conducted on younger, healthier adults. This makes it harder to predict the effects of a given drug on an older person.

In general, older people need lower doses of medication than younger people do. They are more likely to experience side effects, such as confusion, drowsiness, nausea or headaches. Many accidents and falls are the result of such side effects. These side effects may even mimic symptoms of other diseases; confusion due to medication may be mistaken for the onset of Alzheimer's disease, for example. Improper management of medications is a leading reason for nursing home placement of older adults (Fig. 14-2). Be certain that your doctor rules out the possibility of side effects or drug interactions before treating your loved one for any new symptoms.

Many older adults are medicated for multiple long-term conditions at the same time (Fig. 14-3). They may be seeing several doctors; each may be prescribing medications without the knowledge of the others. Be certain that every doctor your loved one sees is aware of every medication that he is taking, including over-the-counter medications, herbal remedies, and vitamin supplements. This will enable his doctors to ensure that the same medication is not prescribed more than once in different forms (a brand name and generic form, for example) and make it easier to avoid adverse drug interactions.

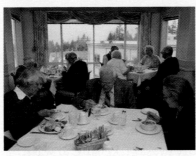

Fig. 14-2. Improper management of medications is a leading reason for nursing home placement of older adults.

Forms of Medication

The general term "pill" is used to refer to any solid medication taken by mouth (Fig. 14-4). This includes tablets, capsules, and lozenges. Pills may be dissolved in the mouth, chewed, or swallowed whole with a drink. For those that are to be swallowed, follow the directions on the label to make sure the liquid used is appropriate. Water is usually best;

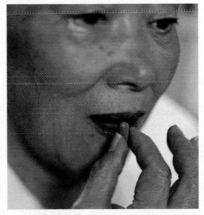

Fig. 14-3. Older adults may take medication for multiple long-term illnesses at the same time.

milk and some juices can reduce the effectiveness of some medications.

Most tablets can be either chewed or swallowed. Time-release tablets are designed to release medication evenly over a specific period of time to maintain a certain level of the drug in the body; they should not be crushed or chewed. Tablets should be swallowed with plenty of liquid to avoid discomfort in the throat. Some are coated to prevent stomach irritation.

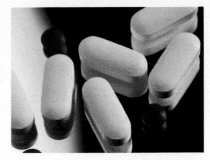

Fig. 14-4. A pill is any solid medication that is taken by mouth.

Capsules may come in the form of hard gelatin shells containing powder or softer gelatin pods containing a liquid. Either of these can be easily swallowed with a liquid. In some cases, if preferred, they can be opened and the contents can be mixed with food or drink for consumption. Ask your doctor or pharmacist before doing this.

Lozenges, also called "troches," are designed to dissolve slowly in the mouth. They are typically used for directly medicating the mouth or throat. They should not be used by people who have trouble swallowing, as there may be danger of choking.

Liquid medications are useful for those who have trouble swallowing pills and are less likely to irritate the stomach. Some liquids must be shaken well before use; read the label for specific directions. Do not use a liquid medication if it has changed color or turned cloudy. To keep the label clean and easy to read, pour with the label facing upward. For accurate measurement, use a measuring spoon or a clear plastic medication measuring cup that can be found at a pharmacy, not a household spoon (Fig 14-5). More potent liquid medications will come with a calibrated dropper to ensure accuracy in measurement. Liquid medications can be taken with water or other clear liquids to minimize un-

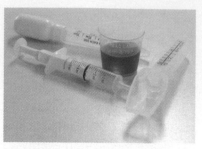

Fig. 14-5. Accurate measurement is important when using liquid medications.

pleasant taste; serving cold can also mask the flavor.

Some liquid medications, called suspensions, contain medication in a suspended rather than a dissolved form. These medications must be shaken thoroughly (8 to 10 times) before use to ensure that the correct dosage is given.

Sublingual medications are placed under the tongue to dissolve, producing a quicker response than drugs that pass through the stomach first. Nitroglycerin is administered in this way. Buccal medications are placed between the cheek pouches and the gums to achieve the same rapid effect as sublingual medications.

Transdermal patches are applied to the skin to release medication slowly and steadily over a designated period of time. These patches work well for people who may forget to take their medication or when periodic dosage is not effective in treating a problem. It is important to remember to remove the old patch before applying a new one and to rotate locations to avoid skin irritation. Check that the patch is securely affixed after bathing or sleeping, and make sure to apply the medicated side of the patch to the skin.

Eye drops and ointments are applied directly to or around the eye (Fig. 14-6). They may be used to treat long-term conditions, such as glaucoma, or to cure infections, treat irritation, or lubricate dry eyes. Make sure to wash hands before use and do not touch anything with the applicator tip. Keep the lid tightly closed when not in use.

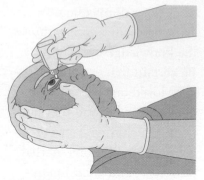

Fig. 14-6. Eye drops are applied directly into the eye.

Ear medications, or otics, are dropped into the ear canal. These are typically used to treat infection or to remove excess wax in the ear. For wax removal, make sure the drops do not run out of the ear until they have been given time to work. For comfort, warm the bottle in your closed hands for a few minutes before use.

Nasal preparations are typically used to treat nasal or sinus congestion and are available over the counter. Overuse of these products can cause them to become ineffective; this is known as a "rebound" effect.

Inhalers are small metal canisters that deliver a measured dose of medicine to help alleviate breathing difficulties (Fig. 14-7). Overuse can reduce effectiveness, especially with over-the-counter versions. Inhalers are used to

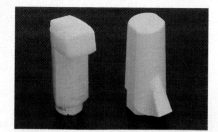

Fig. 14-7. Inhalers are used to ease breathing difficulties.

relieve symptoms of chronic obstructive pulmonary disease (COPD), asthma and other respiratory conditions.

Rectal medications are used to relieve local discomfort or to stimulate bowel movements (Fig. 14-8). They may also be used for pain relief or treatment of nausea for those who cannot take oral medications.

Vaginal medications are used to treat local infection. These may be prescribed, but there are many effective nonprescription treatments available as well.

Topical medications, including ointments, creams and lotions, are used to relieve itching, rashes and infections or other skin conditions. It is a good idea to wear gloves to apply topical medications.

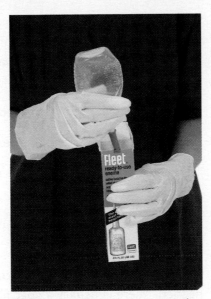

Fig. 14-8. Rectal medications may be used to stimulate bowel movements.

Labeling, Packaging and Storage

Prescription drugs have different labeling requirements from over-the-counter drugs. These requirements can and do change. The guidelines given here are intended only as a general guide for reading and interpreting prescription and over-the-counter drug labels.

GUIDELINES
Drug Labels

Prescription drugs include a package insert that contains detailed information about the drug. This information includes the drug's generic and brand names, all uses that the drug is approved for, side effects and other cautionary statements, a description of how the drug works, how to store it properly, the doses and dose forms available, and how it should be administered.

Not all prescription drug labels will look the same; state laws vary as to what is required to be included. Common label elements include information about the pharmacy, doctor and patient information, the number of refills remaining, the date the drug was prescribed, and directions for proper use, including any special instructions such as shaking before use or storing in the refrigerator (Fig. 14-9).

Companies manufacturing over-the-counter medications assume that people using their products will not be consulting a doctor prior to use. They include detailed information about storage, use, and side effects and other precautions on the label (Fig. 14-10). There is usually more information with greater detail included on a package insert; these inserts should be kept with the medication.

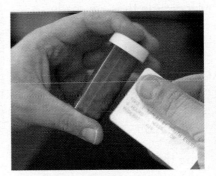

Fig. 14-9. State laws vary as to what is required on prescription labels. Most include doctor and pharmacy information, the number of refills, special instructions, the quantity, and warnings.

Medications 14

Federal law requires child-resistant packaging for both prescription and over-the-counter medication. Those with poor eyesight or arthritis may have trouble opening childproof lids. If this is the case, drugs with regular caps or lids can be requested from the pharmacy.

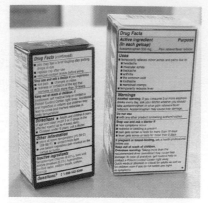

Fig. 14-10. Over-the-counter drug labels may have more detailed information than prescription drug labels.

Before leaving the pharmacy with prescription medication, read the label carefully. Make sure the instructions on the label match the instructions given by the doctor. When medication is being refilled, pharmacies do not always check with the prescribing physician to make sure the instructions and dosages are current. Ask your loved one's doctor to write down changes every time they are made so that you can make sure the labels are current (Fig. 14-11). Do not expect to be able to remember every change in instruction for every medication.

One thing you will find on a prescription drug label will be a schedule for taking the medication. Some medications, called routine medications, are to be taken at

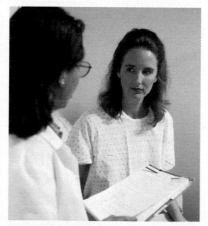

Fig. 14-11. Ask the doctor to write down all changes in medication dosages and instructions.

certain times of the day, such as at bedtime. Routine medications that are taken more than once a day should be spaced as evenly as possible throughout waking hours. Some scheduling abbreviations you may see are:

HS – hour of sleep (time for medication)

BID – take two times a day; for example 9:00 AM and 9:00 PM

TID – take three times a day; for example 9:00 AM, 1:00 PM and 5:00 PM

QID – take four times a day; for example 9:00 AM, 1:00 PM, 5:00 PM and 9:00 PM

Some medications may be designated "PRN," or taken as needed. There is usually a specified limit to the amount that should be taken, such as four times a day or no more than six pills per day. If there is no limit specified on the label, ask the doctor for the maximum safe amount. It is a good idea to keep a written record of how often these medications are taken, especially if there is an increase in use for some reason.

In order to maintain the effectiveness of medications, it is important to store them correctly. This becomes even more important the longer the medicine is stored. Many medications will have specific guidelines for storage on the label or in the package insert, but in general it is a good idea to keep medications in a cool, dry, dark place. The bathroom medicine cabinet, surprisingly, is one of the worst places to store medication. The humidity in the bathroom can make capsules stick together and tablets swell up and break apart.

Some general tips for medication storage are:

- Always read and follow the storage directions on the label.

- Do not store internal and topical medicine in the same place.

- Store medications in a cool, dry place in the original container with labeling intact.

- Do not store medications in the refrigerator unless specifically instructed to do so.

- Store medications away from windows, as exposure to light reduces their potency.

- Keep containers tightly closed.

- Keep medications out of reach of children (Fig. 14-12).

- Do not throw outdated or spoiled medications into household trash accessible to children or pets. Dispose of them by throwing them into the toilet and flushing immediately.

The key to safely managing medications is organization. Keep a complete list of your loved one's medications and when and how they should be taken. To create this list you can use the following ideas:

- Identify and contact all of your loved one's doctors and pharmacies to get a complete record of all current prescription medications.

- Ask your loved one as

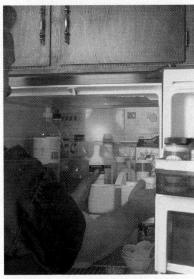

Fig. 14-12. Keep medications out of reach of children.

well as other family members and friends to list all over-the-counter medications she is taking, including vitamin supplements and herbal remedies. Look in all areas of the home where medications are stored to make this list as complete as possible.

- Record any drug allergies and any adverse reactions that she has experienced with any medication.

- Update this information every time there are additions or changes.

The forms at the end of this book will help you organize this information.

Once you have compiled this list, you can schedule the administration of medication. You may want to use a calendar to indicate the times that medication needs to be given, marking them off as they are completed. There are many devices available to make scheduling easier. There are inexpensive organizers that allow you to prepare medications for the day or week in advance (Fig. 14-13). These can help save time and prevent missed or repeated doses of medication.

The following are some general guidelines for assisting with medications:

GUIDELINES

Assisting with Medications

Create a medication schedule using a calendar or one of the

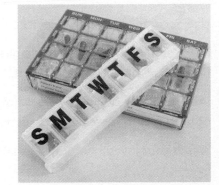

Fig. 14-13. There are many inexpensive devices available to help you organize medications.

forms at the end of this book (Fig. 14-14).

Wash your hands before starting to prepare medications (Fig 14-15).

Prepare the medication in a quiet, well-lighted area free from distractions.

Check that you have the correct medication; make sure the exact quantity prescribed is given at the recommended times.

Check the expiration dates.

Check for discoloration, strange odor, or anything else that is unusual. Do not use any medication that has changed color or turned cloudy.

Do not give medication if you are unable to read the label.

Use accurate measuring devices to prepare doses.

Make sure that your loved one has privacy for taking medications, even pills, if she desires it.

Provide plenty of liquid for swallowing pills; this can be a good opportunity to increase fluid intake.

Watch your loved one until you are sure the medication has been taken.

Keep a written record of any times she decides not to take any medication.

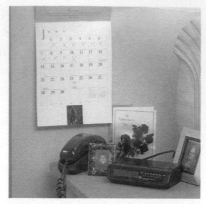

Fig. 14-14. A calendar can help you keep track of when medications have been taken.

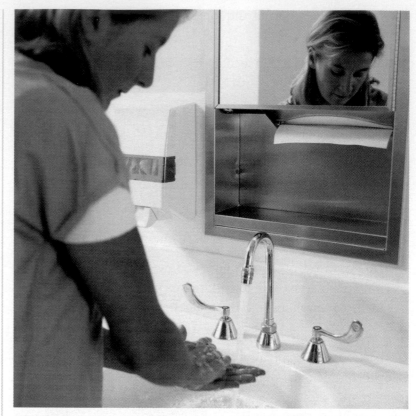

Fig. 14-15. Healthcare workers must wash their hands often, and you should too. Always wash your hands before and after administering medications to your loved one.

Store all containers promptly.

If there are children in the house, store all medications in child-proof containers, especially those stored in the refrigerator.

Do not store different pills in the same bottle.

Wash your hands after medications are administered.

Record the date, time, and dosage immediately after giving medications. Take your medication log on all doctor visits.

If your loved one wants to stop taking any medication, talk to her doctor. Some medications need to be taken for the full time indicated even if symptoms are gone. Others need to be tapered off to avoid harmful reactions. Other medications may need to be adjusted if one is stopped.

Problems with Medication

No medication, prescription or over-the-counter, is completely safe for everyone. To achieve the benefits of medication, we must accept the risk of side effects, allergies, or drug interactions. These may occur shortly after taking medication, or they may take days or even weeks to occur. Some of these may be merely annoying; others may be dangerous, even life-threatening. By being vigilant in the use of medications and keeping an open line of communication with your loved one's doctors and pharmacists, you can maximize the benefits of medications and minimize the risks.

Some common side effects of both prescription and over-the-counter medications include:

- drowsiness
- dry mouth
- headache
- confusion
- nausea
- decreased alertness
- constipation, diarrhea, or incontinence
- loss of appetite
- falls

- depression, lack of interest
- weakness, dizziness
- hallucinations
- anxiety, sleeplessness
- decreased sexual desire
- skin rashes

If any of these occur, do not assume that they are just signs of getting older. Ask your loved one's physician about possible causes.

Another possible problem, especially for older adults who are taking multiple medications, is drug interactions. Both prescription and over-the-counter medications can interact with each other, with food or drink, and even with certain illnesses (Fig. 14-16). These interactions can decrease or alter the effectiveness of the drugs and increase the likelihood of bothersome or dangerous side effects.

A good way to reduce the possibility of problems with drug interactions is to get all of your prescriptions from the same pharmacy. Many pharmacies keep detailed computer records of the medications their customers are taking. Ask your pharmacist to run a scan of your loved one's medications, especially any new ones, to determine if there is any danger.

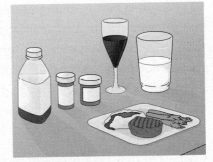

Fig. 14-16. Medications can interact with each other, food, drink, or alcohol.

If you observe any unexpected symptoms or changes, contact the doctor or pharmacist right away. Make sure the event goes onto your loved one's medical record and on your master medications log.

Side effects and adverse reactions are not the only problems that can occur with medications. Listed below are some common problems with medications and how to avoid or address them.

Missed doses: Do not automatically double up the next dose if a medication is missed. Ask your doctor or pharmacist what to do. Often labels will say when to skip and when to take a missed dose.

Wrong dose or wrong medication is taken: Notify your loved one's doctor immediately, even if no ill effects are immediately apparent.

Polypharmacy: Polypharmacy refers to problems caused by taking several different medications at the same time. If doctors are not aware of all medication a person is taking, drugs may be prescribed that will interact with each other. There is also a risk of similar drugs being prescribed or even the same drug being prescribed twice, creating a greater therapeutic effect than intended and increasing the risk of side effects. **Be certain that all doctors are aware of all of the medications that your loved one is taking.** One way to do this is to designate a primary physician and have all other doctors consult her before prescribing medication for your loved one.

Cost: Cost may be a problem in filling or refilling prescriptions (Fig. 14-17). Some people may also take an expensive medication less often than directed to make it last longer. Be sure to tell the doctor if cost is an issue. There may be a less expensive alternative, or there may be other ways the doctor or a medical social worker can help.

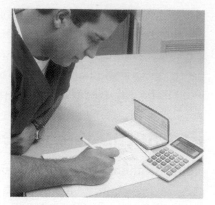

Fig. 14-17. Let your loved one's physician know if the cost of medication is a problem.

Noncompliance: Not all noncompliance with doctors' recommendations is deliberate. Lack of understanding may be the problem; it can also be caused by poor eyesight or poor hearing. Comprehensive, easy to understand, written instructions from the doctor may help. A person may stop taking medication because she is feeling better and thinks she doesn't need it anymore, or because of unpleasant side effects. She may self-medicate symptoms that are actually side effects of other medications she is taking (Fig. 14-18). She may have trouble swallowing pills, or she may simply forget to take the medication.

Noncompliance can be life-threatening, but it can often be corrected if the reason for it is known. Talk to the doctor about any issues that you feel could lead to noncompliance. Also be aware of any conflicts the medication pre-

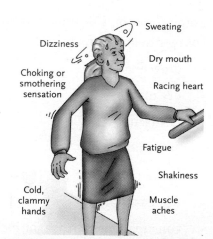

Dizziness
Sweating
Dry mouth
Choking or smothering sensation
Racing heart
Fatigue
Shakiness
Cold, clammy hands
Muscle aches

Fig. 14-18. Your loved one may be medicating symptoms that are actually side effects of other medications.

scribed may have with your loved one's lifestyle. For example, it may make her groggy and reduce her enjoyment of life, or it may require eating more meals a day than she usually eats. Make sure that she has the opportunity to ask questions and give feedback about the medications prescribed.

Common Over-the-Counter Medications

Many older adults self-medicate in addition to taking prescription drugs. Some of the over-the-counter medications commonly used by older adults include:

- Antacids neutralize stomach acid to ease heartburn or stomach upset (Fig. 14-19). Digestive problems may occur if too much stomach acid is neutralized. Antacids can cause a "rebound" effect if overused. Excessive use may indicate a problem beyond stomach upset. Some prescription drugs should not be taken with antacids.

- Pain medications (analgesics) are used to reduce pain, fever and sometimes inflammation. They can be harmful if used in excess of recommended dosage.

- Cough and cold medications should be approved by a doctor before use.

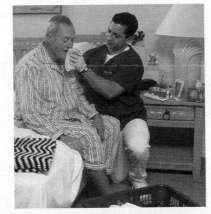

Fig. 14-19. Many older adults take antacids to relieve heartburn or stomach upset.

- Eyedrops and washes that are available over the counter should not be used at the same time as prescription eye medication.

- Laxatives can have a rebound effect if overused. If possible, it is better to treat constipation with diet or with laxatives that are as similar to dietary fiber as possible.

- Topical antiseptics, antibiotics, and antifungal agents are used to treat minor skin irritation and prevent infections. Report any allergies and rashes to the doctor.

The *Physician's Desk Reference* is a great resource for information about medications. See the "Resources" section at the end of this chapter for more information.

Saving Money on Prescription Medications

For some people, the cost of medical prescriptions is a large burden on their financial resources. This can be a dangerous situation, particularly if it causes noncompliance with a plan of treatment. If cost is an issue, be sure to let the doctor know; there may be help available that you are not aware of.

One possible source of assistance is Medicare. Some assistance with prescription drugs is available under the Medicare Prescription Drug Improvement and Modernization Act of 2003. Visit www.medicare.gov to find out if your loved one is eligible. Check back with the site often; this is new legislation and there are likely to be changes.

Many states also have drug programs, and some pharmaceutical firms have their own programs for the elderly.

Learn about drug purchasing programs available to you. Your physician should direct you to these. Some other ways to save money on prescription drugs include:

- Contact your local Area Agency on Aging to find out if your state has any prescription assistance programs for people over 65.

- Ask the doctor if there is a generic or older drug that will achieve the same therapeutic effect at a lower cost.

- When a new drug is prescribed, ask for a trial size rather than an entire thirty-day supply. If the drug does not work out, you will not have paid for medication that will not be used.

- Doctors often have samples of medications that they are given by drug companies. Ask if these are available, especially for new or very expensive medications.

- Buy maintenance drugs that will be taken for a long period of time in larger quantities; a 90-day supply is cheaper per unit than a 30-day supply.

- Order maintenance drugs by mail; they may be cheaper than at a drugstore because there is less overhead.

- Shop around; call pharmacies to find out prices for various medications. Ask if they offer discounts for senior citizens.

Be sure that your loved one does not share prescription medications with others or alter dosages of prescribed medications in an attempt to save money. This is unsafe and can negate any benefit your loved one receives from the medication.

Physicians can be some of the greatest allies in helping an older adult to maintain his or her dignity and quality of life. It is essential to communicate effectively with them. Below are guidelines to help you get all of the information you need and some questions to ask when a new medication is prescribed.

- Schedule a consultation with a healthcare professional to go over the plan of treatment. Bring your master list and all medication bottles. Be sure to tell the doctor about any over-the-counter medications being used, as well as caffeine or alcohol (Fig. 14-20).

- Take notes as you listen and ask for any printed material the doctor can give you. Repeat instructions to make sure you have understood.

- Find out why each medication is needed and how much it is expected to improve your loved one's condition.

- Tell the doctor about any allergies or food sensitivities.

Get the following information about any new medication:

- the brand name and the generic name of the drug

- what it will do

- how often it should be taken

- how long it will take before the drug begins to work

- potential side effects and what to do if they occur

- potential drug interactions and what to do if they occur

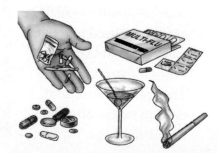

Fig. 14-20. Make sure your loved one's doctor knows about all drugs that are being used, including caffeine and alcohol.

- what to do if a dose is missed

- the risks of overdose and what to do if this occurs

- how long the medication is to be taken

- any risks associated with not taking or not finishing the medication

- if any other approaches, such as diet or stress reduction, could help the problem

- the lowest effective dose

- a prescription written to include the purpose of the medicine (This will ensure that the information is put on the label.)

- if your loved one should avoid any foods, cigarettes or alcohol while taking the medication (Fig. 14-21)

- if medicine must be taken with a meal, with water, with milk, etc. (Fig. 14-22)

- whether it is safe to drive while taking the medication

- whether exposure to sunlight should be avoided

- any written material available about the drug

- how the medication should be stored

- how to dispose of the medication properly if it expires or if treatment is discontinued or completed

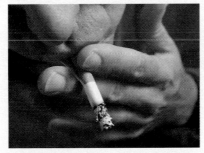

Fig. 14-21. Ask the doctor or pharmacist if any foods, cigarettes or alcohol should be avoided with any medication. (Photo courtesy of Frederick Miller, MD.)

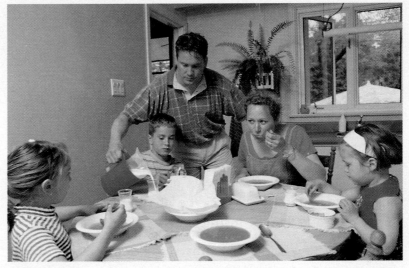

Fig. 14-22. Ask the doctor or pharmacist if medication should be taken with or without food.

It is helpful to establish a relationship with the pharmacy where you purchase prescriptions (Fig. 14-23). Many pharmacies have sophisticated computer systems that keep track of all of the medications that their customers are taking. They also have information regarding food and medication allergies. This can be helpful in averting potentially dangerous situations. Other information that your pharmacist can provide includes:

- How to properly store medications, such as those that need to be refrigerated or kept away from light

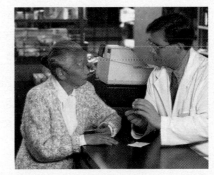

Fig. 14-23. The pharmacist is a good source of information about prescription and over-the-counter medications.

- How to administer medications, such as those that must be shaken before use or taken with water

- When the medication expires

- How long before or after a meal a medication should be taken

- Information on drug interactions

Before leaving the pharmacy, look at the package for any signs of tampering such as broken seals, open or damaged wrappings, or puncture holes. Check the label to make sure it is the correct drug and that the instructions are clear.

When interacting with the pharmacy, you can do the following:

- Even if you competitively shop for prescriptions, choose one main pharmacy to keep track of all of the prescription and over-the-counter medications your loved one is taking. This will help to catch any potentially dangerous situations.

- Ask the pharmacist to write out any complicated instructions clearly on the label.

- If the medication you receive is different in size, shape or color from what you have received before, ask the pharmacist to explain the difference.

- Ask the pharmacist to include both generic and brand names on medication bottles. Use of the generic name helps facilitate communication with and between health professionals.

Resources

The FDA has the latest information on labeling and packaging requirements for prescription and over-the-counter medications. The website also has information about medical devices such as pacemakers and hearing aids. There are also links to report a problem with a product or to comment on proposed FDA regulations.

U.S. Food and Drug Administration
5600 Fishers Lane
Rockville MD 20857-0001
Tel: 888-INFO-FDA (888-463-6332)
www.fda.gov

The Physician's Desk Reference is a comprehensive resource for information about prescription and over-the-counter medications, including herbal medicines and nutritional supplements. It is available in libraries, bookstores, and on the web at www.pdrhealth.com.

Medical Appointment Record

Family and patient medical history

_____

_____

_____

_____

Questions to ask the doctor

_____

_____

_____

_____

Treatment recommendations

_____

_____

_____

Hoped for outcome of recommended treatments

_____

_____

_____

Complications if treatment is not followed

_____

_____

_____

_____

Family and caregiver feedback to treatment

Will it be done?_____

Are there any modifications needed to the treatment?

_____

_____

Actions taken on treatment recommendations

_____

_____

_____

Results of treatment or recommended tests

_____

_____

Coordinating Care Form

Monday Tuesday Wednesday Thursday Friday Saturday Sunday   Date ____/____/____

---

morning
Caregiver

_____

afternoon
Caregiver

_____

evening
Caregiver

_____

night
Caregiver

_____

bed time

_____

breakfast

time _____   Caregiver _____

menu _____

assist feeding _____

lunch

time _____   Caregiver _____

menu _____

assist feeding _____

dinner

time _____   Caregiver _____

menu _____

assist feeding _____

bathing and dressing

time _____   Caregiver _____

Medications
List times, medication and who will assist.

_____

_____

_____

_____

_____

Appointments for today
List appointments and who will drive/assist.

_____

_____

_____

_____

Coordinating Care Weekly Planning Form

Use this form to keep track of your loved one's appointments and activities. Add each event to the appropriate day, then fill in the time of the event and the name of the caregiver responsible for driving or other assistance.

Week of ___/___/___ through ___/___/___

Monday _____

_____

_____

_____

Tuesday _____

_____

_____

_____

Wednesday _____

_____

_____

_____

Thursday _____

_____

_____

_____

Friday _____

_____

_____

_____

Saturday _____

_____

_____

_____

Sunday _____

_____

_____

_____

Home Safety Checklist

General

- ○ Is the home familiar to the person being cared for?
- ○ Is the home accessible for a wheelchair, cane, or walker?
- ○ Are there working smoke alarms where needed?
- ○ Are smoke alarms tested regularly?
- ○ Are the batteries charged?
- ○ Are all houseplants in the home nonpoisonous?
- ○ Are all stoves and furnaces located a safe distance away from window curtains?
- ○ Are appliances that are rarely used disconnected when not in use?
- ○ Are all unused electrical sockets plugged closed?
- ○ Are any firearms stored unloaded and in locked cases?
- ○ Are firearms and ammunition stored separately?
- ○ Are emergency telephone numbers, including poison control, posted near the telephone?

Stairs and Halls

- ○ Does the home have stairs?
- ○ Will your loved one need to use them?
- ○ Are banisters secure?
- ○ Do the edges of treads have non-skid tape on them?
- ○ Is the carpeting or covering on the stairs secure?
- ○ Are stairways free of toys, tools, and other clutter?
- ○ Are there gates at the top of stairs?
- ○ Are the head and foot of stairs free of throw rugs?
- ○ Is there adequate light on stairs?
- ○ Is lighting controllable at both ends of stairs?
- ○ Does the home have changes in floor levels?
- ○ Are the hallways clear and free of clutter?
- ○ Are the hallways free of throw rugs?
- ○ Is there adequate lighting in hallways?
- ○ Is lighting controllable at both ends of halls?
- ○ Are there places where handrails are needed along walls?
- ○ Are any existing handrails secure?

Living Areas

- ○ Are the floors free of clutter?
- ○ Have any throw rugs been removed?
- ○ Have all space heaters been removed?
- ○ Are all electrical cords safely trailed so as not to cause falls?
- ○ Have all unsafe electrical cords been replaced or removed?
- ○ Are electrical cords kept out from under rugs, doors, and furniture?
- ○ Is lighting adequate?
- ○ Are mobility aids available for getting on and off chairs if needed?
- ○ Is there any extra furniture that could be removed?
- ○ Has any shaky or unstable furniture been repaired or removed?
- ○ Is furniture free of rough spots and splinters?
- ○ Is all seating secure?
- ○ Do all chairs have armrests?
- ○ Is furniture secure from slipping on the floor?
- ○ Does the fireplace screen fit properly?
- ○ Is the fireplace extinguished before bedtime?

Bedroom

- ○ Are mobility aids available for getting in and out of bed if needed?
- ○ Is furniture placed to allow clear passage between bed, door, and bathroom in the dark?
- ○ Is there a light switch or lamp within easy reach from the bed?
- ○ Is there a night light to illuminate the room?
- ○ Does the bed have siderails to prevent falls if needed?
- ○ Is smoking in bed prohibited?
- ○ Are dresser drawers kept closed when not in use?

Home Safety Checklist *continued*

Bathroom

- ○ Is the bathroom door labeled if needed?
- ○ Are mobility aids available for getting on and off the toilet if needed?
- ○ Are there grab bars for the toilet?
- ○ Is there a raised toilet seat for easier standing?
- ○ Are mobility aids available for getting in and out of the tub if needed?
- ○ Are there grab bars for the tub?
- ○ Does the tub floor have a non-slip surface?
- ○ Are mobility aids available for getting in and out of the shower if needed?
- ○ Are there grab bars for the shower?
- ○ Is a shower chair available if needed? Are the feet secure?
- ○ Are all hazardous cleaning supplies and chemicals locked away?
- ○ Are all medications stored out of reach and in childproof containers?
- ○ Are all electrical fixtures and appliances located and used at least an arm's length away from the sink, tub, and shower?

Kitchen

- ○ Are all hazardous cleaning supplies and chemicals locked away?
- ○ Is there a fire extinguisher?
- ○ Is it charged?
- ○ Is it in a place that is reachable in case of a stove fire?
- ○ Are all frequently used kitchen items, including potholders, within reach?
- ○ Is all storage appropriately labeled?
- ○ Are matches and lighters kept out of reach?
- ○ Are knives and other sharp items kept out of reach?
- ○ Do can openers leave safe, non-sharp edges on cans and lids?
- ○ Are panhandles kept turned away from stove edges?
- ○ Is floor clean, dry, and free of spills?
- ○ Are all gas burners properly adjusted and free from heat?
- ○ Are flames of gas burners protected from drafts?
- ○ Are flammable materials kept at a safe distance from stove?
- ○ Are all electrical fixtures and appliances located and used at least an arm's length away from the sink and stove?
- ○ Is clothing worn while cooking or in the kitchen free of loose sleeves and other dangling material?

Porch, Yard, and Garage

- ○ Are all outdoor railings and banisters secure?
- ○ Are all steps and walkways kept free of snow and ice?
- ○ Is the yard free of holes, broken glass, tools, and clutter?
- ○ Are dangerous chemicals such as antifreeze and insecticide kept locked away in their original containers?
- ○ Are wires and low fences brightly painted or marked to make them easily visible?
- ○ Are wells, cisterns, and pits securely covered?
- ○ Is there a safe storage area for bicycles and other small vehicles?

Prescribed Medication Information

Brand name _____

Generic name _____

Reason prescribed _____

_____

Date started ___/___/___ Date stopped ___/___/___

Form of medication (circle one)   liquid   tablet   capsule   patch

Color and shape of medication _____

Should the pill be cut or crushed? (circle one)   yes   no

_____

Common side effects and warnings _____

_____

_____

Prescribing Doctor's name _____

Phone _____

Specialty _____

Pharmacy name _____

Phone _____

Address _____

When and how often to take _____

_____

_____

Dosage to be taken and maximum dosage per day _____

_____

_____

What should/should not be taken with, i.e. meal, coffee _____

_____

_____

Duration _____

_____

What to do if a dosage is missed _____

_____

Notes _____

_____

_____

_____

_____

Prescribed Medication Schedule

List all medications taken and the times and conditions under which they should be taken.

Time *or* day	Name of medication	Dosage	How to take

Medication List for Doctor Visit

List all prescription, over-the-counter, herbal, homeopathic and recreational drugs.

Name of medication	Dosage quantity	How often	Duration	Reason for taking	Notes

Index